CARNIVORE UNCOMPLICATED

The No-Nonsense Guide to Metabolic Health, Fat Loss, Fitness, and Food Freedom

By Clinton Scitern

Copyright

Carnivore Uncomplicated

The No-Nonsense Guide to Metabolic Health, Fat Loss, Fitness, and Food Freedom

For permission requests, write to the author at: cs@domesouthpublishing.com

To get the most out of this book, grab the companion journal, Carnivore Uncomplicated 30-Day Reset Journal, and use it to track your food, energy, cravings, sleep, movement, and progress during your reset.

1st edition: May 2026. Printed in the United States of America.

Disclaimer

This book is for general informational purposes only. It is not medical advice and is not intended to diagnose, treat, cure, or prevent any disease. The author is not a doctor or licensed healthcare professional. The information presented is based on the author's personal experience, independent research, observation, and practical use of the principles discussed in this book. Before making changes to your diet, medications, supplements, exercise routine, or overall health plan, consult a qualified healthcare professional, especially if you have a medical condition, take prescription medication, are pregnant or breastfeeding, or have a history of disordered eating. Individual results will vary. The author and publisher are not responsible for any injury, loss, adverse reaction, or outcome resulting from the use, misuse, or interpretation of the information in this book.

Stay Connected. Join the Carnivore Uncomplicated Newsletter

Get simple carnivore tips, practical health lessons, book updates, and no-nonsense guidance from Clinton Scitern, author of Carnivore Uncomplicated.

www.clintonscitern.com

YouTube channel:

www.youtube.com/@clintonscitern

Before you close this book and step back into real life, I want to give you something simple to help you start.

Download your **FREE QUICK START BONUS** here:

www.carnivoreuncomplicated.com

Dedication

This book is for the person who is tired, hurting, and wondering why nothing has worked.

For the one who has tried to do everything right and still feels stuck in a body that doesn't feel like their own. For the one who was told to eat less, move more, and try harder, and is still stuck, still tired, still hungry.

This book is for you.

You are not weak. You are not lazy. You are not broken. Maybe you were just handed the wrong information for too long. My hope is that this book helps you find your way back to better health, one simple step at a time.

Stay the course.

CONTENTS

A Quick Glossary

Before we get started, here are two words you'll see throughout the book. Knowing what they mean up front will make the rest of the read a lot smoother.

Carnivore

Carnivore is a simple, animal-based way of eating built around meat, eggs, fish, and animal fats. It cuts out plant foods, processed foods, sugar, seed oils, and modern additives so the body has fewer things to react to. The goal is to give the body the most usable nutrition possible while making digestion, energy, and metabolism easier to manage. At its core, carnivore isn't about restriction, it's about going back to the foods humans have leaned on for strength, survival, and health for generations.

Ketovore

Ketovore is a high-fat, animal-based diet that blends the ancestral roots of carnivore with the metabolic flexibility of keto. The main focus is still on fatty meats and other animal products, but it leaves room for a strategic, minimal amount of select fermented foods, low-toxicity whole-food plants, and whole-food fats. It's an easier on-ramp into an animal-based lifestyle, mostly animal foods, but with enough variety that meals don't feel boxed in. The aim is to keep the body burning fat for fuel while giving you more options along the way.

PREFACE

Welcome to the Exit Strategy

If you're holding this book, chances are you're tired of trying things that just don't work. Maybe you've counted calories, tracked points, choked down salads, bought all the "healthy" foods, and logged your miles on the treadmill, and you still ended up tired, inflamed, hungry, and carrying weight you can't shake. That isn't a personal failure. It might just mean you were handed the wrong instructions.

For decades, we've been told meat is dangerous, fat is the enemy, and the road to health runs through grains, plants, low-fat everything, and a cabinet full of processed food. But look around. People aren't getting healthier. Obesity, diabetes, depression, bad sleep, low energy, and chronic disease are everywhere you turn.

This book is a way out. It's about questioning the food rules you were raised on and swapping them for something a whole lot simpler: eat real animal-based food, cut the junk, and give your body the chance to do what it was built to do.

What's ahead is about more than a diet. It's about taking your health back. Doing something different from the crowd isn't always easy. But if what the crowd is doing clearly isn't working, maybe it's time to stop following it.

Welcome to the tribe.

— Clinton Scitern

INTRODUCTION

We're living in a time when health information is everywhere. Doctors, medications, food labels, fitness trackers, sleep trackers, calorie apps, smartwatches, podcasts, videos, endless advice telling us how to eat, move, sleep, and live. By all logic, we should be the healthiest people in history. We're not.

Instead, a lot of us are overweight, exhausted, inflamed, sick, and frustrated. Obesity, insulin resistance, poor sleep, digestive trouble, low energy, chronic inflammation, for many people, these have quietly become part of everyday life. And the advice only gets more complicated. Eat this. Avoid that. Count this. Track that. Snack often. Fear fat. Trust fake foods. Use substitutes. Then somehow blame yourself when none of it works.

That raises an uncomfortable question. What if the problem isn't you at all? What if the problem is the advice itself? What if your body isn't struggling because something is wrong with you, but because it's being forced to survive in a world it was never built for? A world full of processed food, seed oils, sugar, fake ingredients, constant snacking, artificial light, poor sleep, and almost no real movement.

For me, that question stopped being theory. It got personal. I hit a point where the usual advice just wasn't working anymore. My body was throwing up warning signs, sleep apnea, premature ventricular contractions, metabolic numbers heading the wrong way, and a bone-deep sense that I wasn't just tired, I was worn down. I was doing most of what we're all told to do, and my health kept sliding anyway. That was my turning point. I didn't need another slogan. I needed to actually understand the problem. What came next wasn't just a change in food, it was a return to the basics my body had been missing: real food, better movement, sunlight, proper sleep, and a simpler way of living.

That's where this book starts. The carnivore framework isn't a fad, a rebellion, or something you have to take on faith. It's a return to the basics. Strip the diet down. Make it simple enough that you can actually see what's helping and what's hurting. Eat foods that give your body the nutrients it needs in a form it can actually use. Cut the noise that keeps your hunger, cravings, digestion, and energy bouncing all over the place. Then pay attention to what happens.

That's why this book is about more than meat. It's about questioning what you were taught about food, hunger, and what your body supposedly needs. It's about rebuilding the foundation, how you eat, how you move, how you recover, how you sleep. The body doesn't heal from one thing alone. Food matters, but so do movement, rest, light, and recovery.

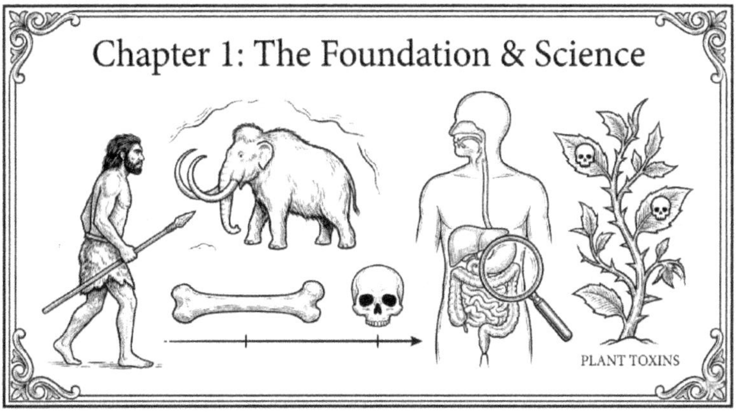
Chapter 1: The Foundation & Science
PLANT TOXINS

CHAPTER 1

THE FOUNDATION & SCIENCE

The carnivore diet often gets called extreme because it pushes back against most of what we've been taught about nutrition. But looked at from another angle, it isn't extreme at all, it's simple. It pulls eating back to the basics and asks one honest question: what does the human body actually need to function, heal, and stay strong?

That's why carnivore makes sense to so many people. We're living in a world packed with processed carbs, seed oils, fake ingredients, addictive foods, and a flood of confusing health advice. One person says one thing. The next person says the opposite. Carnivore cuts straight through that confusion. It strips out the foods that tend to trigger cravings, bloating, inflammation, digestive trouble, blood sugar swings, and weight gain, and zeroes in on animal foods that are rich in protein, fat, and nutrients the body can actually use.

My own transition into this way of eating wasn't smooth or easy. Like a lot of people, I dealt with cravings, electrolyte issues, and the mental tug-of-war of walking away from foods I'd eaten my whole life. But once I pushed through the adjustment, something shifted. My hunger settled. The cravings faded. My energy felt steady instead of riding a rollercoaster. Food stopped running my thoughts the way it used to.

To understand how a diet this simple can create such a big change, we must start with the foundation. This chapter walks through the main idea behind carnivore: why animal foods matter, why nutrient density and bioavailability are a big deal, why certain plant compounds cause problems for some people, and why a lot of common nutrition advice deserves a second look before this way of eating really clicks.

THE CORE PHILOSOPHY

At its heart, carnivore is built on one question: what does the human body actually need to survive, repair itself, and get healthy?

Strip away food marketing, diet trends, cultural habits, and confusing nutrition advice, and the answer gets a lot simpler. The body needs the right building blocks. It needs usable energy. And it needs a stable environment, one where its hormones aren't being thrown off constantly by junk food, sugar, processed oils, and overeating. Carnivore is built on the idea that animal foods deliver these things in one of the most direct, concentrated, and usable forms there is.

The first pillar is essentiality. In nutrition, some things are essential, meaning your body can't make them on its own, so you have to get them from food. Essential amino acids are needed to build and repair the body. Essential fatty acids are needed for normal health and function. These aren't optional. Without them, your body can't maintain muscle, repair tissue, regulate hormones, heal, or even stay alive.

Carbohydrates are a different story. Your body can use them, but they aren't essential in the same way. There's no known dietary requirement for carbs because your liver has a backup system called gluconeogenesis. In plain English, your liver can make the glucose (blood sugar) your body needs out of protein and fat byproducts. It doesn't mean nobody should ever eat them. It just means carbs are optional, while protein and fat are foundational.

That difference matters, because modern nutrition tends to flip the order. People are pushed toward grains, fruit servings, snacks, fiber, and carbs, while a lot of them aren't getting enough quality protein, animal fat, or the key vitamins and minerals that animal foods deliver. Carnivore turns that order right-side up. It starts with what the body actually needs and clears out what isn't required, so the body finally gets a chance to settle down.

The second pillar is bioavailability. That's just a fancy word for how well your body can absorb and use the nutrients in a food. A food can look healthy on a label and still not deliver much your body can actually use. This is where animal foods have a major edge. Meat, eggs, seafood, and organs contain nutrients in forms the body recognizes, absorbs, and puts to work.

Take iron, for example. The iron in red meat is called heme iron, and the body absorbs it far more easily than the iron found in plants. Liver contains vitamin A in its active form, called retinol. Plant foods contain a different form that has to be converted first, and some people don't convert it well. Animal foods also deliver B12, zinc, creatine, carnosine, taurine, and complete protein, all in highly usable forms.

Plant foods can be more complicated. Many of them contain fiber, compounds that can reduce mineral absorption, or chemicals that can irritate the gut in some people. These are often called antinutrients, things like oxalates, lectins, phytates, and other plant defense chemicals. That doesn't mean every plant is toxic. It doesn't mean nobody can tolerate plants. It just means plant foods aren't always as simple as we've been told. From a pure efficiency standpoint, animal foods are usually easier for the body to break down, absorb, and use with less friction.

That idea of reducing friction is a big part of carnivore. Your body is always working. It must digest food, absorb nutrients, regulate blood sugar, balance hormones, repair tissue, and handle stress. The more complicated the diet, the more variables it has to juggle. Modern diets are stacked with processed foods, seed oils, sauces, sweeteners, starches, snacks, and addictive combinations of fat, sugar, and salt. These foods confuse hunger, ramp up cravings, and make it a whole lot easier to overeat.

That leads to the third pillar: hormonal simplicity. Carnivore removes most of the foods that drive cravings and overeating. When food is highly processed, heavily flavored, and engineered to be hard to stop eating, hunger stops being about what your body needs. It becomes driven by stimulation, habit, comfort, and reward. Cravings get louder. Fullness signals get quieter. The brain starts chasing flavor and pleasure instead of true nourishment. That's not a willpower problem; it's a food environment problem.

By simplifying food choices and cutting out the processed stuff that overstimulates the brain, the body gets a chance to calm down and reset. Hunger becomes easier to read. Fullness becomes easier to feel. Ghrelin (the hunger hormone) and leptin (the fullness and energy-balance hormone) can start working in a less chaotic environment. For a lot of people, that's the biggest shift they notice. Food stops feeling like a constant battle and starts being what it was always meant to be, fuel, nourishment, and recovery.

This simplicity also makes it easier to hear what your body is telling you. When the diet is stripped down to a small group of nutrient-dense animal foods, the feedback gets clearer. If bloating, fatigue, skin issues, cravings, digestive problems, or inflammation start to improve, that's useful information, your body is saying something. If you add a food back later and the symptoms come back, that signal is much easier to catch. In a diet full of sauces, grains, sweeteners, fibers, oils, spices, and processed ingredients, it's nearly impossible to know what's causing what. In a simple diet, the message gets through.

The goal isn't to turn carnivore into a religion. It's not to pretend everyone has to eat exactly the same way. The goal is to recognize that the body usually works better when it gets what it needs in a form it can actually use, while removing the foods and habits that mess with hunger, cravings, digestion, and metabolism. Carnivore is a lot like cleaning out a messy room, you take out what doesn't need to be there so you can finally see what matters.

At its core, this philosophy is about trusting biology over food trends. The body doesn't care about marketing, labels, slogans, or popular opinion. It cares whether it's getting the raw materials it needs. It cares whether it can absorb those nutrients. It cares whether your hormones are being supported or constantly disrupted.

The core philosophy of carnivore comes down to this: give the body what it truly needs, in a form it can use, and clear out the noise that throws off hunger, fullness, digestion, and metabolism.

The Evolutionary Argument

Why do many researchers believe meat played a major role in human evolution? Because the evidence doesn't come from just one place. It shows up in our bodies, our digestion, our energy needs, and the bones and tools left behind by ancient humans.

Humans developed large brains that demand a lot of energy. At the same time, compared to great apes, we have smaller digestive systems. That combination matters, because both the brain and the gut are energy-expensive to maintain. The Expensive Tissue Hypothesis lays it out simply: as the human brain grew bigger, the body had to make tradeoffs somewhere else. One of those tradeoffs was likely a smaller gut and a shift toward foods that were more energy-dense and easier to digest.

Gorillas and other large primates can pull a lot of energy out of fibrous plants, but their guts are built for that work. They also spend huge chunks of the day chewing and processing massive amounts of plant material. Humans aren't built like that. We're not designed to sit around all day eating leaves and fermenting fiber in a giant gut. Our digestive system fits much better with a higher-quality, more nutrient-dense diet.

Our stomach acid tells part of the story too. Human stomach acid sits at a pH of roughly 1.5 to 2.0, stronger than most primates and closer to animals that regularly eat meat or scavenged food. Strong acid helps break down animal foods and may also help kill off harmful bacteria. That doesn't prove humans are strict carnivores, but it does back up the idea that meat has been an important food for us for a very long time.

The archaeological record makes the case stronger. Scientists can study ancient bones for clues about what people were eating. One method looks at nitrogen levels in bone collagen. In simple terms, higher nitrogen levels usually mean a person or animal ate higher on the food chain. Studies of Neanderthals and ancient humans often show nitrogen levels that place them high up, sometimes close to, or even above, large meat-eating animals from the same region.

That doesn't mean every ancient human ate only meat. Humans are adaptable. We can survive on a wide range of foods depending on the environment. Some groups leaned more on plants. Some leaned on fish. Others depended heavily on big animals, fat, marrow, and organs.

But here's the bigger point: animal foods weren't a small side dish in human history. For long stretches of time, especially during the Ice Age period known as the Pleistocene, animal foods appear to have been central. Meat, fat, marrow, organs, and seafood likely supplied the calories and nutrients humans needed to grow big brains, travel long distances, reproduce, build strength, and survive in harsh environments.

That's the real evolutionary argument. It isn't that every human population ate the exact same diet. It's that the human body carries the fingerprints of a species that leaned heavily on animal foods to become what it is today.

These lines of evidence don't prove that every modern person must follow a carnivore diet. But they do make one thing hard to ignore, meat wasn't a small footnote in human evolution. It was one of the main drivers.

THE PLANT PARADOX

Most of us were raised on the idea that plants are always healthy and eating more vegetables always equals better health. But that idea is a bit too clean.

Plants are living things too. They have their own way of surviving. Since plants can't run, fight, bite, or hide, many of them protect themselves with chemicals instead. Seeds, leaves, stems, roots, and skins can carry compounds that help the plant fend off insects, animals, mold, or being eaten.

It doesn't mean every person reacts badly to plants. It just means plants aren't automatically harmless for everyone. They're chemically active, and pretending they have no effect on the body ignores how nature actually works.

This matters because modern nutrition tends to treat all plant foods as automatically good. But some plant compounds can interfere with digestion, reduce mineral absorption, or irritate the gut and immune system in certain people. A healthy person with strong digestion may breeze through these compounds. Someone dealing with autoimmune issues, digestive problems, kidney stone risk, chronic inflammation, or a damaged gut may not.

The carnivore argument isn't that every plant is poison. The better way to put it is this: plants contain defense compounds, and some people feel a lot better when those compounds are reduced or removed.

Take lectins. Lectins are proteins found in many plant foods, especially beans, grains, and some nightshades. Some lectins can be reduced by soaking, fermenting, sprouting, and proper cooking. That's part of why traditional cultures took the time to prepare beans and grains carefully before eating them.

But poorly prepared lectin-rich foods can cause digestive trouble in some people. Certain lectins can also interact with the gut lining and the immune system. The strongest, most honest claim isn't that lectins are destroying everyone's gut. It's that lectins are active compounds, some are harder to digest, and in sensitive people they may contribute to gut irritation.

Oxalates are another example. They show up in foods like spinach, almonds, rhubarb, beets, and several other plants. In some people, oxalates can raise urinary oxalate levels and may increase the risk of kidney stones.

Phytates are another one worth understanding. Phytic acid lives in grains, seeds, legumes, and nuts. It binds to minerals like iron and zinc and makes them harder for the body to absorb. That's part of why a plant food can show minerals on the nutrition label that your body never fully gets. This matters most in diets that lean heavily on grains and legumes while including very little animal food. Again the point isn't that phytates are wrecking everyone's health. It's that plant nutrition isn't always as straightforward as the label makes it look.

Then there are glycoalkaloids. These are natural compounds in potatoes and other nightshades. In high amounts, they can be toxic. For most people eating properly stored and prepared potatoes, the risk is low. But the bigger lesson still stands; plants make chemicals that affect the body, and some people are more sensitive to those chemicals than others.

Plants aren't morally good or bad, they're complex. Some people tolerate them well, others don't. If your gut is inflamed, your joints ache, your skin reacts, your digestion is unreliable, or your immune system feels constantly stirred up, dialing down plant defense compounds may help you see whether they're part of the picture.

A carnivore elimination approach can be useful precisely because it removes a lot of those variables at once. It gives the body a simpler environment. Then you can see what improves, what doesn't, and what foods seem to cause issues if you add them back later.

Chemical	**Found In**	**The Problem**
Lectins	Legumes, nightshades (tomatoes, peppers), grains	Sticky proteins that can bind to the gut lining, potentially contributing to intestinal

		permeability ("leaky gut") and immune activation.
Oxalates	Spinach, kale, almonds, rhubarb	Sharp, crystal-like compounds that may accumulate in tissues, contributing to kidney stones or joint pain in susceptible individuals.
Phytates	Grains, seeds, nuts	Mineral chelators that bind zinc, calcium, iron, and magnesium, reducing absorption.
Glycoalkaloids	Potatoes, eggplant	Naturally occurring plant toxins that can disrupt cell membranes and

		promote inflammation in sensitive individuals.

Common Myths

To succeed with carnivore, you have to unlearn a lot of nutrition advice that's been repeated for years. Just because something has been said often doesn't mean it's always true.

Many common nutrition "rules" are either exaggerated, misunderstood, or only true in certain situations. People are told fiber is always necessary, red meat is always dangerous, and fruit is the only real source of vitamin C. But when you actually look closer, none of these claims are as clean as they sound.

Carnivore challenges these ideas because it forces you to ask better questions. Instead of swallowing every nutrition rule whole, you start looking at how the body actually works and what the evidence really shows.

- **Myth 1: "You Need Fiber to Stay Regular"**

This is one of the most repeated claims in nutrition. Most people have heard it their whole life, if you want to poop regularly, you need more fiber. But that idea is too simple.

Fiber isn't a required nutrient like protein, fat, vitamins, or minerals. Your body doesn't digest most of it. It mainly adds bulk to stool, changes its texture, and affects how fast food moves through the gut. For some people, especially people eating a mixed diet, certain kinds of fiber may help digestion. But that doesn't mean more fiber is always better, and it doesn't mean fiber is required for everyone to have normal bowel movements. The honest version is this: fiber may help some people, but it's not a universal requirement. So basically if you're eating enough fat you should not be constipated even while eating zero fiber.

On carnivore, bowel movements often change. Stool volume usually drops because animal foods are highly digestible and leave less waste behind. In plain English: your body uses more of the food, so less comes out. Less stool doesn't automatically mean constipation. If you're not in pain, not bloated, and not straining, going less often might just mean your diet is producing less waste. That's different from having a problem.

The principle is simple. Constipation isn't always caused by a lack of fiber. It can come from poor gut motility, dehydration, low salt, low fat intake, stress, medication, or just the body adapting to a new way of eating. If the real issue is one of those, piling on more bulk won't fix it. In some people, it'll make things worse.

The better lesson: bowel regularity doesn't follow one rule for everyone. It depends on what you eat, how much waste that food creates, how hydrated you are, how much fat and salt you're getting, and how your own digestive system responds.

- **Myth 2: "Red Meat Causes Cancer and Heart Disease"**

This one gets treated like proven fact, but the truth is messier. A lot of the fear around red meat comes from studies that look for patterns in large groups of people. These studies can show that two things happen together, but they can't prove that one caused the other.

That matters, because surveys suggest that people who eat more red meat often have other habits that affect their health. Some smoke more, drink more alcohol, exercise less, carry more body fat, eat more fast food, or eat more processed food in general. Surveys also suggest that people who avoid red meat, on the other hand, are also more likely to exercise, avoid smoking, and stick to other health habits. So, when a study says red meat is "linked" to disease, that doesn't automatically mean red meat caused the disease. It means the evidence is weaker and messier than the headlines suggest.

There's also a big difference between fresh red meat and processed meat. A steak, a roast, or plain ground beef isn't the same as processed meat served with a bun, fries, seed oils, sauces, and a sugary drink. That distinction gets brushed aside far too often.

Some research shows stronger links between processed meat eaten with other processed foods and health problems than between fresh, unprocessed red meat and health problems. A fresh steak and a fast-food meal aren't the same thing inside your body. The better claim is that the case against fresh, unprocessed red meat is much weaker than most people have been led to believe, and your overall diet should mean more to your health.

- **Myth 3: "You'll Get Scurvy"**

This is one of the first things people throw out when they hear about carnivore. They assume that if you don't eat fruit, you'll automatically get scurvy. But that's too simple.

A real vitamin C deficiency causes scurvy. That part is true. What people often miss is that vitamin C needs can shift depending on the rest of the diet. Fresh animal foods also contain small amounts of vitamin C, especially organ meats (also called offal) and fresh meat that hasn't been overcooked. Offal just means the edible organs and parts of an animal, liver, heart, kidney, tongue, and tripe (the stomach lining).

Some researchers have pointed out that fresh meat and organs can supply enough vitamin C to help prevent scurvy. That doesn't make vitamin C unimportant, it means fruit isn't the only possible source. There's also an idea floating around in low-carb circles that sugar and vitamin C may interact in ways that affect how the body uses vitamin C. The better point is that vitamin C needs may not look the same on every diet, and skipping fruit doesn't automatically mean scurvy is around the corner, but this is where you have to be careful.

There have been cases of scurvy in people eating very limited diets, including meat-heavy diets that lacked freshness, variety, or enough nutrients overall. The safer conclusion is this: scurvy isn't guaranteed on carnivore, especially when fresh meat and organs are part of the picture. But it isn't something to wave off either. Food quality, freshness, and variety within animal foods still matter.

The real lesson behind these myths isn't that every mainstream nutrition claim is false. Some of them have truth in them, but they're often exaggerated or treated as if they apply to everyone the same way. Fiber may help some people and bother others. Fresh red meat isn't the same as processed junk food. Vitamin C deficiency isn't a problem on a will rounded animal-based diet, but it can't be dismissed carelessly either.

SUMMARY OF CHAPTER 1

Chapter 1 lays out the idea that carnivore isn't just another diet trend. It's a return to the basics. Instead of starting with food rules, diet labels, or popular opinion, it starts with one simple question: what does the human body actually need to survive, repair, and function well?

The point isn't that everyone must eat the exact same way. The point is that the body has clear priorities. Protein and fat are essential, your body needs essential amino acids and essential fatty acids to build, repair, regulate hormones, and stay alive. Carbohydrates can be used for energy, but they aren't required in the same way, because the body can make the glucose it needs through gluconeogenesis.

We also looked at the role animal foods played in human evolution. Humans developed large brains that demand a lot of energy. At the same time, compared to many other primates, we have smaller digestive systems. That combination makes a lot more sense once you understand that humans leaned heavily on high-quality, nutrient-dense animal foods like meat, fat, marrow, organs, and seafood.

That doesn't mean every ancient human ate only meat, but it does show that animal foods weren't a small side dish in human history. They were a major part of how humans survived, developed, and became what we are.

The chapter also pushed back on the common idea that plant foods are always harmless. Plants are living things, and many of them protect themselves with natural chemicals, lectins, oxalates, phytates, and glycoalkaloids. These compounds don't affect everyone the same way. In some people, they can irritate the gut, reduce mineral absorption, trigger immune reactions, or add stress to the body.

That's one reason a carnivore elimination approach can be useful. By removing many plant compounds and processed ingredients at once, the body has fewer things to react to. It becomes easier to see what improves, what stays the same, and what foods may be causing problems if you add them back later.

Finally, the chapter addressed some of the biggest myths about meat-based eating, the claim that everyone needs fiber, the claim that red meat automatically causes cancer and heart disease, and the claim that a carnivore diet guarantees scurvy.

The truth is more nuanced than the slogans. Fiber may help some people and bother others. Fresh red meat isn't the same as processed junk food. And scurvy isn't guaranteed on an animal-based diet, especially when fresh meat and organs are part of the routine, though food quality and variety still matter.

The main lesson of Chapter 1 is simple: carnivore isn't about blindly rejecting everything you were taught. It's about questioning it. It's about starting with what the body truly needs, removing what may be causing problems, and paying close attention to the results.

Chapter 2: What to Eat & Sourcing

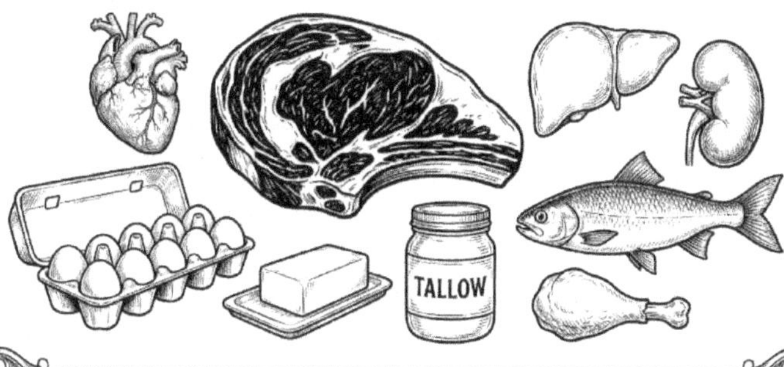

CHAPTER 2

WHAT TO EAT & SOURCING

Chapter 2 is where carnivore stops being just an idea and starts becoming something you can actually follow. Theory matters, but theory alone doesn't change your health, food does. Your results come from what you put on your plate, how consistent you are, and whether your choices match what your body needs right now.

This chapter is about cutting through the confusion. Instead of guessing what to eat, you need a clear order of importance. Some foods should be the foundation. Some are useful extras. Some work well for one person but cause problems for another. The goal is to replace random food choices with a simple system that makes sense.

The first thing to get clear on is that carnivore isn't just one diet, it's a range of approaches. Some people need to be very strict, especially in the beginning. Others do better with a version they can follow for years. Some can handle a little more flexibility without losing progress. The right version depends on your body, your symptoms, your metabolism, and your goals.

This matters because not everyone is starting from the same place. Someone dealing with serious food reactions, gut issues, autoimmune symptoms, or major metabolic problems may need a much stricter approach. Someone who mainly wants to lose fat, improve energy, or simplify their eating may not need that same level of restriction. Some people need a hard reset. Others need a steady long-term plan. Others do well with a more flexible animal-based approach.

From there, this chapter builds out the food hierarchy. Ruminant meat sits at the top because it's one of the most stable, reliable foundations there is, beef, bison, lamb, deer, elk. Organ meats can add powerful nutrition in small amounts. Eggs and dairy may be useful for some people, but they aren't automatic staples for everyone. And fat isn't the enemy, on carnivore, fat is one of your main fuel sources.

By the end of this chapter, you should be able to look at your plate and know whether the food is supporting your body or working against it. The goal isn't just to ask, "Is this carnivore?" The better question is, "Is this helping me get the result I need?"

The Spectrum of Carnivore and the Hierarchy of Sourcing

One of the biggest mistakes people make with carnivore is thinking there's only one correct way to do it. There isn't. Carnivore is better understood as a spectrum, stricter on one end, more flexible on the other. The version you need depends on where your health is right now.

If someone is metabolically unhealthy, inflamed, reactive, or dealing with serious symptoms, a stricter version usually makes sense in the beginning. If someone is already healthier, more stable, and less reactive, they may handle more flexibility without losing the benefits. So, the better question isn't "Is carnivore right?", it's "what version of carnivore is right for me right now?"

That difference matters because people have different goals. Someone trying to calm autoimmune symptoms, fix their digestion, or figure out serious food reactions isn't in the same place as someone who just wants to lose body fat, think more clearly, or stop eating junk. Both may benefit from an animal-based approach, but they don't need the same level of strictness.

Some people need a hard reset. Others need a simple plan they can follow long-term, while others do well with a more flexible animal-based version that keeps them stable without going overboard. Most people don't stay at one level forever. As the body changes, symptoms improve, and tolerance becomes clearer, you may move from one level to another. That's normal.

These levels aren't meant to become labels or identities, they're tools. The point isn't to pick one version and defend it like a religion. The point is to use the simplest version that gets you the result you need.

NAVIGATING THE THREE TIERS

The carnivore spectrum breaks down into three main tiers. Each tier has a purpose. Each can be useful. But each one works best when you choose it honestly, based on your body and your goals, not your ego.

- **Level 1 — The Lion Diet: The Ultimate Elimination**

This is the strictest version of carnivore. It's also the clearest version for people who need to figure out what their body may be reacting to. The Lion Diet usually means ruminant meat, salt, and water only. Ruminant meat means beef, lamb, bison, deer, and elk. No eggs, no dairy, no pork, no chicken, no seafood, no seasonings beyond salt, and no plant foods at all.

This level is usually best for people dealing with serious issues, metabolic syndrome, autoimmune symptoms, major digestive problems, chronic skin issues, stubborn inflammation, or a long history of reacting poorly to many different foods. It isn't meant to be fancy. It's meant to be simple, strict, and clear.

When the body is highly sensitive, too much variety actually makes things harder. The Lion Diet strips out almost everything except the most basic foods. That gives the body a chance to calm down and makes it easier to see what's helping and what's hurting. If symptoms improve while you're eating this way, that tells you something important. If symptoms come back when you add a food back in, that tells you even more.

The idea is simple: remove eggs, dairy, pork, poultry, spices, sweeteners, and plant foods, and you've removed many of the most common food triggers all at once. That's what makes the Lion Diet one of the strongest tools for figuring out what your body can and can't handle.

This doesn't mean everyone has to eat this way forever. For most people, it's a starting point, not a life sentence. But for someone whose health is too unstable for guessing, it can be the clearest place to begin.

- **Level 2 — Carnivore: The Sustainable Baseline**

This is the level where most people will spend most of their time. Standard carnivore includes animal meats, seafood, eggs, and animal fats, with ruminant meats as the foundation, beef, lamb, bison, deer, and elk should still form the core. This level is still zero-carb or very close to it but gives you more variety than the Lion Diet.

It fits people who want fat loss, better body composition, steadier energy, clearer thinking, better appetite control, and long-term metabolic health. Simple enough to keep cravings and food confusion low, but flexible enough to actually live with. For a lot of people, this is the sweet spot, strict enough to work, but not so strict that it feels impossible to maintain.

The advantage of standard carnivore is that it opens up more options without dragging back the full confusion of plant-based eating. Eggs can be convenient and nutritious. Seafood adds important minerals. Pork and poultry can add variety, though they usually work best as secondary options to ruminant meats if your main goal is health optimization.

This is the level where most people learn how to build an animal-based lifestyle that actually works in real life.

- **Level 3 — Ketovore: The Flexible Framework (a.k.a. Dirty Carnivore)**

This is the most flexible version. Ketovore starts from the standard carnivore foundation but allows a few selected extras, heavy cream, aged hard cheeses, dry spices, occasional low-carb plant foods. For some people, that may include extra virgin olive oil, avocado, olives, fermented or unfermented low-carb vegetables, or pickles. For others, it just means using seasonings or including small amounts of dairy without issues.

Ketovore is usually best for people who've already built a strong foundation. Their metabolism is stable, cravings are under control, digestion has improved, and they know what foods they tolerate. It can also help people who find strict carnivore hard to maintain socially, professionally, or mentally over the long haul. But this level has one big danger: drift.

A little flexibility can work for some people, but it can also be a slippery slope. A few pickles turn into fruit. Fruit turns into "clean carbs". Clean carbs turn into weekend cheat meals. Before long, the old habits are back.

Ketovore only works when animal foods stay the foundation. The extras must stay optional. They can't take over the diet. If the added foods start driving cravings, overeating, inflammation, or poor choices, they're no longer helping.

How to Choose Your Starting Point

If your body feels inflamed, sensitive, unpredictable, and full of symptoms, start stricter. If your main goal is fat loss, better body composition, appetite control, and simpler eating, standard carnivore is usually enough. If you already have good metabolic health and mainly want an animal-based way of eating with a little more flexibility, ketovore may be the right fit.

The biggest mistake is starting too loose when your body clearly needs more structure. Your body gives feedback, but only if the message is clear enough to hear. Someone dealing with metabolic syndrome, severe eczema, autoimmune symptoms, bloating, migraines, and joint pain probably doesn't need "moderation" in the beginning. They need clarity.

On the flip side, someone who already feels good, has stable energy, and is metabolically healthy doesn't need to stay at the strictest level forever. The goal isn't to be as strict as possible just to prove a point. It's to use the smallest amount of restriction needed to get healthy and stay healthy.

The Hierarchy of Sourcing

Once you understand the different levels, the next question is where your food comes from. What you eat matters first. Where it comes from matters second. Both matter, but they don't matter equally.

This is where a lot of people get stuck trying to be perfect. They think if they can't afford grass-fed, grass-finished, pasture-raised, regenerative, local, organic everything, then they can't do carnivore correctly. Not true.

Switching from processed food to meat is the biggest upgrade. That matters far more than switching from regular grocery store meat to expensive specialty meat. A regular ribeye from the grocery store is still a far better choice than cereal, a vegan protein bar, fast food cooked in seed oils, or a processed snack. That said, food quality does matter when you have the money and access for it. There's a simple order of importance.

First, prioritize ruminant meats, beef, lamb, bison, deer, and elk. These should be the foundation because they provide strong nutrition and reliable fat.

Second, when your budget allows, buy the best quality you can reasonably afford. Grass-finished and pasture-raised options may have some advantages in fat quality, nutrients, and how the animals were raised.

Third, use pork and poultry strategically rather than making them the center of the diet, especially if they're conventionally raised.

Fourth, treat eggs and dairy based on how your body responds. Don't assume they're harmless just because they're animal foods. Some people do great with them. Others don't.

The rule is simple: don't let perfect stop you from starting.

The best meat is the meat you can afford, cook, and eat consistently in place of junk. If that means regular ground beef from the grocery store, start there. If that means buying larger cuts in bulk or choosing cheaper fatty cuts instead of expensive steaks, do that. You can upgrade food quality later. Just don't delay progress because you can't afford the perfect version on day one.

PROGRESS OVER PURITY

In the end, carnivore isn't one single diet. It's a framework. It ranges from the strictest version (the Lion Diet) to the more flexible version (Ketovore), with standard carnivore sitting in the middle as the best long-term baseline for most people.

The skill is knowing where you belong right now. Not where someone online tells you to be. Not where your ego wants you to be. Where your body actually needs you to be. The right version of carnivore isn't always the strictest version, it's the version that gives your body enough clarity to heal and enough consistency that you can actually stick with it.

THE BIOLOGY OF MEAT: RUMINANTS VS. MONOGASTRICS

At first glance, a pork chop and a ribeye look like two versions of the same thing, meat. But inside the body, they're not quite the same. The animal you eat matters because different animals digest food differently, and that affects the kind of fat stored in their meat. This is important on a carnivore or animal-based diet because you're not just eating meat for protein, you're often using animal fat as one of your main fuel sources. That means the quality of the fat matters.

The main difference is between ruminant animals and monogastric animals. Ruminants include cows, sheep, goats, bison, deer, and elk. These animals have a specialized digestive system with multiple stomach compartments. They can ferment grass and other fibrous plants before those nutrients become part of their body. Because of that digestive system, ruminants transform much of the fat they eat before it gets stored in their meat. That makes their fat more stable, and it also means their meat is usually less affected by feed quality than meat from animals like pigs and chickens.

That doesn't mean feed doesn't matter, it does. Grass-fed beef and grain-fed beef can differ in omega-3 fats, antioxidants, and overall fat quality. But the gap usually isn't as dramatic as it can be with pork or poultry. In simple terms, cows don't store dietary fat as directly as pigs and chickens do. That's one reason beef stays a fairly reliable staple food, even when the animal wasn't raised in a perfect system.

This consistency is exactly why ruminant meat should be the foundation of a carnivore diet. Beef, lamb, bison, deer, and elk provide high-quality protein, stable fat, heme iron, zinc, B vitamins, and other nutrients the body uses well. They're predictable, nutrient-dense, widely available, and reliable. Ruminant meats aren't the only useful animal foods, but they're usually the strongest foundation.

Monogastric animals are different. Pigs and chickens have a single-chambered stomach, more like humans. Because they don't have the same digestive system as ruminants, the fat in their bodies is more directly shaped by what they eat. If pigs and chickens are fed a lot of corn, soy, or other feeds high in polyunsaturated fats, more of those fats end up in their meat and fat. This is especially true with omega-6 linoleic acid. It's also why the quality of pork, chicken, and eggs can swing more depending on how the animals were raised and what they were fed.

This isn't about pork and chicken being bad, that would be too simple. The point is that their fat is more sensitive to feed quality. In commercial farming, that usually means pork and poultry can carry more polyunsaturated fat than beef or lamb. Eating pork or chicken occasionally probably isn't a major issue. But if you're using animal fat as your main source of calories every day, the type of fat matters more. In that case, ruminant fat is usually a cleaner and more stable fuel source than large amounts of pork fat or chicken skin from conventionally fed animals.

This also teaches an important lesson about sourcing. Higher-quality pork, poultry, and eggs can be much better when the animals are raised on better feed. Since pigs and chickens are more affected by what they eat, their quality can swing up or down more dramatically. That means quality matters more with monogastric animals than with ruminants. Beef is more forgiving. Chicken, pork, and eggs are less forgiving.

On a carnivore diet, this hierarchy matters because animal foods aren't a side dish, they're the diet. If most of your calories come from animal fat, then fat quality isn't a small detail. It's central. The simplest rule: make ruminant meat the backbone of your diet. Use pork, poultry, eggs, and other animal foods as secondary options based on tolerance, quality, and goals. When fat becomes your main fuel, the biology of the animal matters. Ruminants provide the most reliable foundation.

Organ Meats: Nature's Multivitamin

Most modern people think organ meats are weird, outdated, or unnecessary. That's mostly a cultural reaction, not a biological fact. For most of human history, people prized organ meats because they were some of the most nutrient-dense parts of the animal. Today, people spend money on vitamins, powders, fortified foods, and supplements while ignoring the foods that naturally contain many of those same nutrients in a form the body can use. That's why organ meats deserve respect again.

Muscle meat is a solid foundation, especially from ruminant animals like beef, lamb, bison, deer, and elk. But organs bring something different to the table. They're far more concentrated in certain vitamins and minerals. You don't need to eat large amounts, in some cases, eating too much is actually a bad idea. The value of organ meats comes from using them wisely. A small amount can deliver a lot of nutrition that muscle meat alone doesn't.

Beef liver is the clearest example. Liver is loaded with vitamin A, vitamin B12, copper, folate, riboflavin, and other key nutrients, which is exactly why it should be treated with respect. Liver is powerful because it's concentrated. Many people do better with small servings once or twice every week or two rather than eating large portions all the time.

Beef heart plays a different role. It doesn't carry the same wide range of nutrients as liver, but it's known for being rich in CoQ10, which helps the body produce energy at the cellular level. Heart is also easier for many people to eat because it tastes more like a dense, rich steak than liver. For people who are nervous about organ meats, heart is often a good place to start.

Bone marrow is different from both. It's valued more for its rich fat and traditional food role than for being loaded with vitamins. It may also contain interesting compounds that affect the immune system, but the research isn't strong enough to call it a miracle food. Think of marrow as a nourishing ancestral fat source, not magic.

One reason organ meats matter in an animal-based diet is that they bring back the old nose-to-tail way of eating. Modern people gravitate toward familiar cuts, steaks, roasts, ribs, ground beef. Traditional people prized the organs and fattier parts because they understood those parts were deeply nourishing. They also wasted far less of the animal.

Of course, none of this matters if you can't make yourself eat them. The "ick" factor is real. Most people weren't raised eating liver, heart, or marrow, so pretending it's easy for everyone isn't helpful. Start small. Mix a little liver or heart into ground beef. Use it in burgers, meatballs, or meatloaf. Ask a butcher for a custom blend if possible. Most people find that when organ meats are mixed into regular ground meat in small amounts, the taste is much easier to handle.

Another option is using very small pieces of frozen liver to avoid most of the taste. Some people do this, but raw organ meat needs to be handled carefully. Food safety matters. Sourcing matters. For most people, the safer, more practical option is to cook organ meats properly and use small amounts consistently.

Perfect sourcing helps if you can afford it, but it isn't required to benefit. A small amount of regular grocery store liver still contains a serious amount of nutrition. Don't let perfection stop you from making progress. Waiting until you can buy the perfect grass-finished, regenerative, local, boutique organ meat is often just another excuse to delay action. Your body doesn't care about food status. It cares about usable nutrition.

The bigger lesson is simple: organ meats are tools, not commandments. Some people do great eating them regularly. Some only need liver or heart once in a while. Others prefer blends, pâté, or capsules. The form matters less than the principle. Organ meats add concentrated nutrition that supports a meat-based diet. Even small amounts make the overall diet stronger.

DAIRY & EGGS

Muscle meat and organ meats are the foundation of carnivore. Eggs and dairy are a little more complicated. They're animal foods, and they can be nutrient-dense, easy to prepare, and enjoyable. But they can also cause problems for some people. Some folks do great with eggs and dairy. Others notice stalled weight loss, skin flare-ups, stuffy nose, bloating, digestive trouble, cravings, or symptoms that don't improve until eggs or dairy are removed. That's why eggs and dairy shouldn't be blindly defended or automatically rejected.

Not every animal food behaves the same way in the body. Meat is usually simple and predictable. Eggs and dairy have more variables. Eggs contain different proteins that some people may react to. Dairy contains fat, lactose, whey, casein, and other compounds that affect people very differently. The real question isn't, "are eggs and dairy good or bad?", it's, "do eggs and dairy work for my body right now?"

THE INCREDIBLE, POLARIZING EGG

Eggs are an impressive food. Affordable, easy to cook, easy to carry, and packed with nutrition. The yolk is the richest part, it carries choline, fat-soluble vitamins, healthy fats, cholesterol, and a long list of important nutrients. The white is mostly water and protein, including ovalbumin, ovomucoid, ovotransferrin, lysozyme, avidin, and others.

But eggs can be a problem for some people. They're one of the more common food allergens, especially in sensitive individuals. Most of the trouble usually comes from the egg white, not the yolk. Egg white proteins are more likely to trigger reactions in people who are sensitive. Raw egg whites can create another issue too, a protein called avidin can bind to biotin (a B vitamin). That's mostly a concern when someone eats a lot of raw egg whites. Cooking makes eggs easier to digest and can reduce some of the reaction potential.

That's why some people do well with whole eggs. Some do better with mostly yolks. Others discover that eggs are one of the hidden foods keeping their symptoms alive. The yolk is usually the most nutrient-dense part and often the better-tolerated part. The white is still useful protein, but more likely to cause issues in sensitive people.

Sourcing matters too, but the labels can be misleading. Words like "cage-free" and "free-range" don't always mean what people assume. "Pasture-raised" usually means the chickens had more outdoor access and a better shot at eating a more natural diet. Pasture-raised eggs may contain more omega-3 fats, a better omega-6 to omega-3 balance, and more natural color compounds called carotenoids. Not every nutrient changes the same way, but the main point is simple: better-raised chickens usually produce better eggs.

The Dairy Dilemma

Dairy is where a lot of people get tangled up, because it looks like carnivore but doesn't always act like meat in the body. Milk is made to help a young animal grow. That means it isn't just a basic food, it's growth food. It contains lactose, whey, casein, bioactive compounds, and hormone-signaling substances. In plain language, dairy is an active food. It can affect the body in stronger ways than people realize.

One reason dairy can be tricky is that it can raise insulin, especially because of whey and certain milk proteins, even when the dairy isn't high in carbs. Whey protein, in particular, may stimulate insulin more than casein in some people. At the same time, dairy isn't automatically bad. The research is mixed. Some people do fine with it. Some may even improve certain health markers with the right types of dairy. Others don't tolerate it well at all. That's why dairy sits in a gray area.

For people trying to gain weight, maintain muscle, or add calories easily, dairy can be useful. Heavy cream, cheese, butter, and full-fat dairy make it easier to eat more. But for people trying to lose fat, control cravings, or calm skin and digestive symptoms, dairy can quietly work against them. The problem isn't always obvious. Some people don't get severe stomach pain or a clear allergic reaction, they notice smaller things: more hunger, stronger cravings, stuffy nose, bloating, acne, skin redness, mucus, or stalled progress.

That's why dairy should be treated as optional. Some people include it with no problem. Others need to remove it to see real progress.

THE 30-DAY ELIMINATION TEST

The best way to know if dairy works for you isn't to argue about it, it's to test it. Everyone's body is different. Some people handle dairy well. Others don't. The cleanest way to find out is to remove dairy completely for about 30 days, then add it back carefully and watch what happens.

When you bring dairy back, pay attention to warning signs. Skin issues like acne, redness, flushing, or eczema may return. Breathing trouble like a stuffy nose, mucus, or congestion may show up again. Digestive problems like bloating, gas, stomach pressure, or feeling heavy after meals may come back. Other signs include joint discomfort, fatigue, stronger cravings, or stalled progress. None of these symptoms prove dairy is bad for everyone, they just tell you whether dairy is working for your body right now.

NAVIGATING THE DAIRY HIERARCHY

If you tolerate dairy well, you still need to understand that not all dairy is the same. Some forms are easier on the body than others. Butter and ghee are usually the easiest because they're mostly fat. Ghee is typically even easier because most of the milk proteins have been removed. Aged hard cheeses are often easier to tolerate than regular milk because much of the lactose is reduced during the aging process. Lactose is the sugar found in milk, and many people don't digest it well.

Fresh milk, soft cheeses, ice cream, and large amounts of cream are more likely to cause problems, especially for people who are sensitive to lactose or milk proteins. Lactose intolerance is common. If dairy bothers you, the answer may be to reduce it, choose low-lactose options, choose lactose-free options, or remove it completely. Don't assume all dairy acts the same in the body.

Low-fat dairy should be treated carefully in a carnivore framework. That doesn't make every low-fat dairy product toxic, the issue is that removing the fat usually makes the food less filling. It also strips away part of what makes full-fat dairy more complete. Low-fat dairy is also more likely to be paired with sweeteners, flavors, and additives. Highly processed cheese products belong even lower on the list. The further dairy moves away from real food and closer to factory-made food, the less useful it becomes.

THE PRACTICAL RULE

Don't let nostalgia, convenience, or loyalty to a diet label decide this for you. Eggs and dairy can be useful, but they aren't the foundation of carnivore the way ruminant meat is. They're extras.

The order is simple. Build your diet around ruminant meat and animal fat. Add eggs if your body handles them well. Test dairy honestly. Choose the simplest forms you tolerate best. If your body clearly does better without eggs or dairy, accept that answer and move on.

Fats: The Primary Fuel

In the modern diet, fat has been blamed for almost everything. People were taught to trim it off, fear it, avoid it, and replace it with low-fat or fake alternatives. On carnivore, that mindset doesn't work. When you cut carbs or keep them very low, fat becomes your main fuel source. It isn't just something added for flavor, it's what your body uses for energy. Your body can still make the small amount of glucose it needs, and over time it can also make ketones for fuel.

In plain language: if you eat carnivore too lean, you're going to feel bad. This is one of the first big mistakes beginners make. They cut the carbs but keep the fear of fat. Then they try to live on lean meat alone. The result is predictable, low energy, constant hunger, poor fullness, irritability, feeling cold, and a sense that something is missing.

Extreme versions of this problem have been known historically as "rabbit starvation" or protein poisoning. It happens when someone eats too much lean protein without enough fat. The body can use protein for repair and structure, but protein isn't meant to be your main energy source on its own. The body also must deal with the waste from breaking down large amounts of protein.

That's why fat isn't optional in this way of eating. Protein gives the body structure. Fat gives the body fuel. Protein helps build and repair tissue. It supports hormones, enzymes, the immune system, and muscle. Fat provides the dense energy needed to keep the body running when carbs are low. If protein is the lumber and steel of the body, fat is the electricity that keeps the system running. When people say they don't feel right on carnivore, the issue often isn't that they cut carbs, it's that they aren't eating enough fat.

THE ANIMAL FAT LIBRARY

Not all fats act the same in the body or when you cook with them. One advantage of animal fats, especially from ruminants like cows, sheep, bison, deer, and elk, is that they're usually more stable than industrial seed oils. That means they tend to hold up better under heat and are less likely to break down during cooking. This matters because on carnivore, fat isn't just extra flavor. It's one of your main fuel sources, so the kind of fat you use matters.

Beef tallow is one of the most useful fats in a carnivore kitchen. It's stable, easy to cook with, and works well for higher-heat cooking. It also has a mild enough flavor that you can use it often without overpowering the food. Because it comes from a ruminant animal, its fat profile is more reliable than fat from animals like pigs or chickens, especially when those animals were raised on conventional feed. In short, beef tallow is dependable, practical, and fits the carnivore framework well.

Suet is another valuable fat source. It's the hard fat found around the kidneys and loins of ruminant animals. Dense, stable, and rich in saturated and monounsaturated fats, including stearic acid. You don't need to overcomplicate the science here. The main point: suet is a strong, traditional animal fat that many people tolerate well. It gives the body a concentrated source of energy and fits beautifully in a meat-based diet.

Butter and ghee are also useful, but they sit in a slightly different category. Butter adds flavor, richness, and fullness to meals, but still contains some milk solids that can burn at higher temperatures. Ghee is butter with most of those milk solids removed, so it handles heat better and may be easier for some people to tolerate. If dairy works for you, butter and ghee can be excellent tools, just not as foundational as beef fat. Think of them as useful additions, not the base of the entire diet.

Lard and duck fat are more complicated. They taste great and can make food more enjoyable, but they come from monogastric animals. That means pigs and ducks store more of the fat they eat directly in their own body fat. If they're fed a lot of corn, soy, or other feeds high in polyunsaturated fats, their fat can carry more omega-6 linoleic acid than ruminant fat usually does. That doesn't mean lard and duck fat are poison, it just means they're better used as secondary fats, not your main fuel. If your goal is a stable, reliable carnivore foundation, ruminant fats like beef tallow and suet should come first.

PROTEIN VS. FAT

You don't need to treat your body like a math problem. You don't need to track every gram forever or turn every meal into a spreadsheet. Once processed foods are gone, most people can read their hunger and fullness signals much better. Still, a simple rule helps; protein is mainly for building and repairing the body, while fat is mainly for energy. Protein helps build muscle, repair tissue, and support hormones and immune function. Fat keeps the engine running, especially when carbs are very low.

If your energy is low, your hands and feet are cold, your sleep is poor, or you feel oddly unsatisfied after eating, the answer probably isn't more protein, it's more fat. A lot of beginners make this mistake, they eat lean meat, avoid carbs, and still fear fat. Then they wonder why they feel weak, hungry, cold, or flat. On carnivore, lean meat alone often isn't enough. The body needs fuel, and in this framework, that fuel usually comes from animal fat.

On the other hand, more fat isn't always better right away. If very fatty meals make you nauseated, cause urgent diarrhea, or suddenly make rich cuts of meat seem disgusting, that may be a sign your digestive system isn't ready for that much fat yet. Early carnivore takes some adjustment. Your bile production, digestion, and meal rhythm may need time to catch up. In that case, don't force huge amounts of rendered fat. Choose fatty cuts you tolerate better, go a little slower, and let your body adapt.

If you're hungry again shortly after eating, the issue is usually one of two things: the meal was too lean, or you simply didn't eat enough. That's why fattier cuts often work better than lean cuts in real life. A sirloin may look cleaner and leaner, but a ribeye usually satisfies better because it gives you both protein and fat in the same meal. In plain language, it gives your body both building material and fuel. That's why fatty meat is often more useful than lean meat for appetite control, steady energy, and long-term consistency on carnivore.

The Symptom	The Adjustment
Low energy or cold hands	Increase your fat intake. Your "engine" is stalling.
Nausea or a sudden aversion to meat	Reduce fat slightly. Your gallbladder may need time to adapt.
Persistent hunger shortly after eating	Increase your total intake. You aren't eating enough.

When in doubt, choose the fattier cut of meat, ribeye instead of sirloin, and eat until you're truly satisfied. Don't stop because an app, a calorie chart, or an old diet rule tells you to stop. Eat slow and stop when your body feels fed, calm, and steady.

A note on sleep: if your sleep feels broken, lighter, or more restless during the first few weeks, don't automatically assume it's because you aren't eating enough fat. Sleep changes can happen during the transition into carnivore. Your body is changing how it uses fuel and how it handles water, salt, electrolytes, and energy. That adjustment can temporarily affect sleep. It doesn't mean the diet is failing. It usually means your body is still adapting, and sleep issues should be addressed directly instead of blamed on one single thing.

THE TRUE ENEMY

If there's one kind of fat that deserves serious skepticism in this framework, it's industrial seed oils, soybean oil, corn oil, sunflower oil, safflower oil, cottonseed oil, and the rest of the family. These oils are high in polyunsaturated fats, especially linoleic acid. Because of their structure, they're more fragile than stable animal fats and more likely to break down during processing, storage, and high-heat cooking.

These aren't traditional whole-food fats. They're industrially refined oils that are now hidden throughout the modern food supply, chips, crackers, salad dressings, sauces, fast food, fried food, frozen meals, packaged snacks, restaurant meals. That's part of the problem. Most people aren't drinking seed oils by the spoonful; they're eating them without realizing it because the oils are baked into ultra-processed foods.

In a diet built around whole animal foods, seed oils are unnecessary. Once fat becomes your main fuel, the question isn't just how much fat you're eating. The better question is: what kind of fat are you asking your body to run on?

Stable ruminant fats, beef fat, tallow, suet, make the cleanest foundation. Dairy fats like butter and ghee work well for people who tolerate dairy. Fats from monogastric animals like pork, chicken, and duck can play a supporting role, especially when the animals are raised well. Industrial seed oils don’t belong in the diet at all.

On carnivore, fat isn't the enemy of health. Fat is the fuel that lets the system run.

SUMMARY OF CHAPTER 2

In this chapter, we moved past the false idea that carnivore is one rigid diet with only one correct version.

Carnivore is better understood as a spectrum. The Lion Diet is the strictest version and gives the most clarity for people who need a serious elimination approach. Standard carnivore is the sustainable baseline where most people will spend most of their time. Ketovore is the more flexible version for people who already have a strong foundation and can handle more variety without sliding back into old habits.

The main lesson: the right version depends on your body, your symptoms, and your goals. The point isn't to chase dietary purity just to prove you're disciplined. It's to use the level of structure your body needs. If your body is inflamed, reactive, and unstable, you may need more precision. If your body is already doing well, you may not need the strictest version forever. The goal isn't purity. The goal is progress you can sustain.

Ruminant meats, beef, lamb, bison, deer, and elk, were laid out as the most reliable foundation because these animals tend to produce a more stable, consistent fat profile than animals like pigs and chickens. Pork and poultry can still have a place, but they usually work best as secondary foods, not the main source of calories. This matters because on carnivore, meat isn't just a protein source. Animal fat often becomes your main fuel, so the type and quality of that fat matter.

We also looked at organ meats and why they strengthen an animal-based diet. Liver, heart, and marrow aren't foods most modern people are used to eating, but they're rich in nutrients and have been valued in traditional diets for a reason. You don't need large amounts. Even small amounts used strategically add nutrition that muscle meat alone may not provide. The lesson is simple: muscle meat builds the foundation, but organ meats make that foundation stronger.

From a fuel perspective, you saw that fat isn't a side issue on carnivore, it becomes the main energy source once carbs are cut or kept very low. Protein and fat have different jobs. Protein is mainly for structure, repair, muscle, hormones, enzymes, and immune function. Fat is mainly for fuel. Eat too lean and you'll feel hungry, cold, tired, irritable, or unsatisfied. Eat enough fat from the right sources and the diet becomes far easier to sustain.

Finally, we dealt with the gray area of eggs and dairy. Both can be useful foods, but neither should be treated as automatically harmless or required. Eggs may work well for some people and trigger symptoms in others. Dairy may help one person maintain weight and calories while quietly stalling fat loss or driving cravings in another. By using elimination, careful reintroduction, and honest observation, you now have a way to judge these foods by results instead of assumptions.

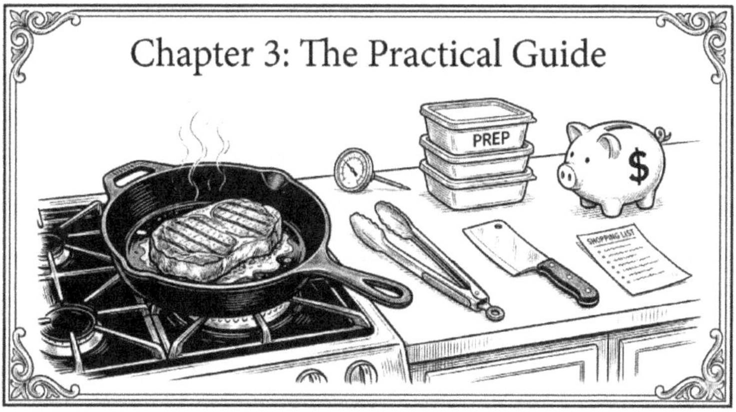
Chapter 3: The Practical Guide
PREP
$
SHOPPING LIST

CHAPTER 3

THE PRACTICAL GUIDE

A carnivore framework can make perfect sense when you read about it and still fall apart in real life if you don't know how to actually live it. Most people don't struggle because the basic idea is wrong. They struggle because they never build the habits and systems that make it doable every day. They don't set up their kitchen in a way that makes cooking easy. They don't learn how to make meat taste good enough to eat day after day. They underestimate the transition period, misread early symptoms, don't get enough salt, don't eat enough food, don't eat enough fat, and make the whole thing harder than it needs to be. Then, when they feel bad or fall off, they blame carnivore instead of looking at the fact that their setup was weak from the start.

Carnivore is simple, but simple doesn't mean automatic. You need a kitchen that makes the diet easier, not harder. You need a few basic cooking skills, so your meals are satisfying instead of dry, boring, and repetitive. You need to understand what the transition can feel like, so you don't mistake normal adjustment for failure. And you need to know how to make this way of eating affordable enough to keep going without feeling like every grocery trip is a financial problem.

I made plenty of these mistakes myself. In the beginning, I tried to push through the adjustment phase on willpower instead of building the right support around me. I underestimated how much salt, hydration, food, and fat mattered. I treated discomfort like something to ignore instead of something to learn from. What follows is the practical roadmap I wish I'd had at the start. It'll show you how to set up your kitchen, cook the food properly, get through the transition more intelligently, and make this way of eating work in normal everyday life.

KITCHEN SETUP: THE CARNIVORE TOOLKIT

You don't need a fancy kitchen, expensive equipment, or professional cooking skills to succeed on carnivore. But you do need a setup that makes cooking meat easy, repeatable, and enjoyable. When most of your meals come from animal foods, preparation matters more than people think. A badly cooked steak, a dull knife, or a pan that never gets hot enough can make the diet feel miserable fast.

This is one of the most overlooked parts of long-term success. People often think discipline is only about mindset, but your environment matters too. If cooking feels annoying, cleanup takes forever, and the food never tastes good, you're going to have a hard time sticking with it. A few good tools make a big difference. They save effort, improve flavor and texture, help keep meat juicy, and make it easier to get consistent results without guessing every time. The goal isn't to build a luxury kitchen. It's to build a simple system that makes eating animal foods easy enough to repeat without overthinking it.

In the carnivore world, skill doesn't come from complicated recipes. It comes from learning the basics, heat, salt, timing, and texture. Once you can sear a steak properly, brown ground beef without turning it gray and watery, cook burgers without drying them out, and make cheaper cuts taste good, the whole lifestyle becomes much easier.

THE ESSENTIALS

These are the basic tools that make the biggest difference for most people eating carnivore. You don't need every gadget on the market, but you do need tools that make cooking meat easier, cleaner, and more consistent. The goal is simple: make it easier to cook good food at home so you're less tempted to fall back into junk, takeout, or convenience food.

THE CAST IRON SKILLET (10–12 INCH)

If you only buy one pan and learn how to use it well, make it a cast iron skillet. It's tough, simple, affordable, and very good at holding heat. That matters because cooking meat well depends on steady heat. A weak pan cools down the moment the steak hits it, and that keeps the meat from getting a good sear. Instead of a rich crust, you end up with pale, watery meat. A hot cast iron skillet gives you what you actually want, a strong sear on the outside and a tender inside.

This is where the Maillard reaction becomes your friend. That's the browning process that creates the crust on meat. It's what makes a steak, burger, or piece of liver taste rich and satisfying instead of plain and boring. Cast iron is excellent for steaks, burger patties, liver, chopped meat, and fatty cuts. It also works well for finishing tougher cuts after slow cooking, crisping fat, and rendering suet or tallow.

A Sharp Chef's Knife

A sharp knife isn't fancy equipment, it's basic equipment. If meat is the center of your diet, you're going to be trimming fat, cutting roasts, slicing steaks, portioning liver, and prepping meat often, a dull knife makes all of that harder. It drags, slips, tears the meat, and turns simple prep into a frustrating job. It's also more dangerous, because you have to push harder to make each cut.

You don't need a drawer full of knives. One good chef's knife or butcher-style knife, kept sharp, will handle most of what you need. If you can trim meat cleanly and cut it into portions without fighting it, you've removed one more problem from daily cooking.

A Large Cutting Board

When meat is the center of the diet, your cutting board matters more than you'd think. A small board creates mess, makes food harder to handle, and turns cleanup into a bigger job. A large cutting board gives you room to work with roasts, ribs, fat trimmings, steaks, and cooked meat without everything sliding off the edge.

Wood, bamboo, stainless steel, titanium, or high-quality plastic can all work as long as they're cleaned properly. I prefer stainless steel or titanium because they're durable, clean, and easy to maintain. The main point is to use a board that's large, practical, and sanitary.

A cutting board with a juice groove is especially useful. On carnivore, the meat juices and rendered fat aren't trash. They carry flavor and fat, and they can be poured back over the food. A good board keeps those juices from running across the counter or onto the floor. It's a small detail, but small details matter when you're repeating them every day.

A Digital Meat Thermometer

A meat thermometer removes guesswork. That matters because guessing is one of the easiest ways to ruin expensive meat. The difference between medium-rare and overcooked can be small, especially with leaner cuts. If you keep pulling steaks too late, drying out burgers, or undercooking thick cuts, a thermometer fixes that problem fast.

This is one of the easiest ways to make your food more consistent. Properly cooked meat tastes better, and food that tastes better is easier to stick with. Carnivore becomes a whole lot harder when every meal is dry, overcooked, or disappointing.

BASIC STORAGE CONTAINERS

This isn't exciting, but it matters. If you buy meat in bulk, cook ground beef ahead of time, save leftover steak, or render your own tallow, you need good storage containers. Glass containers, stainless containers, vacuum-seal bags, or high-quality freezer-safe containers can all work.

The goal is to make meal prep easier. If good food is already cooked, stored, and ready, you're much more likely to stay on plan. If every meal requires starting from zero, excuses multiply. The easier you make the right choice, the more often you'll make it.

THE NICE-TO-HAVES

These tools aren't required, but they can make carnivore much easier. Once the basics are covered, these can save time, improve texture, and make the diet more convenient.

THE AIR FRYER

The air fryer is one of the most useful convenience tools for a carnivore lifestyle. It gives steady heat, takes little effort, and works especially well for foods that taste better with crisp edges and rendered fat. It's great for pork belly, wings, burger patties, sausages, reheated steak, and smaller cuts you don't want to babysit on the stove or grill.

The real value of an air fryer is convenience. It helps you cook quickly without ruining texture. For a lot of people, that means fewer bad decisions when they're tired, busy, or hungry. When food can be ready fast and still taste good, staying consistent becomes easier. If you can, look for an air fryer with a stainless steel or glass basket or tray rather than a plastic-coated one.

The Sous Vide Precision Cooker

A sous vide setup isn't required, but it's a useful tool if you want consistent results. It's especially helpful for making cheaper, tougher cuts of meat taste better than expected. Sous vide cooks food in a water bath at a controlled temperature, which means the meat cooks evenly from edge to edge without accidentally getting overcooked. Thick steaks come out exactly how you want them, and tougher cuts can cook long enough to become tender without drying out.

For someone following carnivore, sous vide can be a strong tool if you care about precision or want to make budget cuts more enjoyable. After the meat is cooked, you finish it with a hard sear in a hot pan or on a grill. That gives you the browned crust on the outside while the inside stays tender and evenly cooked. Done right, even basic cuts can taste like something from a restaurant.

The Slow Cooker or Instant Pot

A slow cooker or Instant Pot is especially useful if you want to make carnivore more affordable. Cuts like chuck roast, brisket, stew meat, oxtail, and short ribs can be tough if you cook them the wrong way, but they turn soft, rich, and satisfying when cooked low and slow or under pressure. These tools let you turn cheaper cuts into meals that are filling, flavorful, and easy to repeat.

This matters because a lot of people think carnivore has to be expensive. It doesn't. You don't need to live on ribeye every day. Tougher cuts are usually cheaper, and when they're cooked properly, they can be every bit as satisfying as expensive steaks, sometimes even better. A slow cooker or Instant Pot makes that possible without requiring much cooking skill.

THE FREEZER

A freezer can become one of the most valuable parts of your carnivore system. You don't need a giant deep freezer to start, but extra freezer space helps. It lets you buy meat in bulk, stock up during sales, store pre-portioned meals, freeze organ meats, and save rendered fat for later. That gives you more control over both cost and convenience.

The freezer also removes pressure. If you always have meat available, you're less likely to panic, order takeout, or grab something that doesn't fit your plan. A stocked freezer means you're prepared before hunger shows up. That matters, because a lot of bad food decisions happen when people are tired, hungry, rushed, and unprepared.

Optional Upgrades That Actually Help

A few extra tools can help, depending on how much cooking you plan to do and how organized you want your system to be.

Kitchen scale. Useful if you want short-term clarity on portion sizes or total intake, especially in the beginning. You don't need to weigh food forever, but it can help you understand how much you're actually eating.

Stainless steel sheet pans and oven-safe racks. Excellent for batch cooking burgers, bacon, wings, roasts, or anything that does well in the oven. They make it easier to cook more food at once and reduce the need to start from scratch every meal.

Tallow jar or fat container. Lets you save rendered fat instead of wasting it. On carnivore, good animal fat is useful. If you cook ground beef, brisket, bacon, or fatty cuts, saving the fat gives you something to cook with later.

Salt cellar or grinder. Small, but useful. Salt is a major part of this way of eating, especially during the transition. Keeping it easy to access makes it more likely you'll use enough.

Vacuum sealer. Very helpful if you buy meat in bulk, freeze portions, or use sous vide often. It protects meat from freezer burn and makes storage cleaner and more organized.

The Real Principle

A good carnivore kitchen isn't about looking fancy. It's about making meat easy to cook, easy to store, and easy to enjoy. That matters far more than having a professional-looking setup. If your kitchen makes the right choice easier, you're more likely to stay consistent.

When your setup is right, the diet becomes easier almost automatically. You stop overthinking every meal. You stop relying on willpower every night. Instead, you create an environment where the default option is a good one. That's the real goal, making the right food easier to choose than the wrong food.

Cooking Mastery: How to Cook Meat Well

A lot of people don't fail on carnivore because the diet doesn't work. They fail because their food becomes boring, dry, and disappointing. When every meal feels like punishment, most people eventually quit. That's why cooking skill matters. If meat is going to be your main food, learning how to cook it well isn't optional, it's part of making this lifestyle work. The difference between a dry, gray steak and a properly cooked steak isn't small. It can be the difference between forcing yourself through the diet and actually enjoying this way of eating.

Good cooking doesn't have to be complicated. It's about understanding the basics. Meat responds to heat, time, moisture, and rest. When you manage those well, even simple food can taste great. Ignore them, and even an expensive steak can be ruined in minutes. The goal isn't to become a professional chef, it's to become skilled enough that your meals taste good, satisfy you, and make it easier to stay consistent.

Carnivore is simple, but cooking skill keeps simple from turning into boring. Once you learn a few reliable techniques, you don't need sauces, side dishes, or complicated recipes to make food enjoyable. You learn how to make the meat itself taste good. That's when this way of eating starts to feel a whole lot more sustainable.

TECHNIQUE A: THE REVERSE SEAR

For thick steaks and roasts, the reverse sear is one of the most reliable methods you can learn. Instead of cooking the outside with high heat first and hoping the inside turns out right, the reverse sear does the opposite. You cook the meat slowly at a low temperature first, then finish it with a hot, fast sear at the end. The result is a more even cook from edge to edge, with a browned crust on the outside and a tender inside.

- **Step one — dry the meat well.** Moisture makes browning harder. If the surface is wet, the pan must burn off that water before it can build a crust. Pat the meat dry with paper towels until the outside feels more tacky than wet. This one step makes a big difference.
- **Step two — season.** Salt the meat generously on all sides. Salt does more than add flavor. It helps pull moisture from the surface, supports browning, and brings out the natural flavor of the meat. If you have time, salt the steak ahead and let it sit uncovered in the

refrigerator. That dries the surface even more and gives you a better crust later.

- **Step three — the low-temperature cook.** Place the meat on a wire rack over a stainless-steel baking sheet and cook it in a low oven, around 250°F, until the internal temperature is about 10 to 15 degrees below where you want it to finish. This slow stage gives you control. It helps the meat cook evenly instead of ending up overcooked on the outside and undercooked in the middle.
- **Step four — the sear.** Heat a skillet with tallow or ghee until it's very hot and just starting to smoke. Then sear the meat for about 45 to 60 seconds per side, sometimes less depending on the thickness of the meat and how hot the pan is. The goal isn't to keep cooking the inside, it's to build a crust fast. If the pan is hot enough, it won't take long.
- **Step five — the rest.** Let the meat rest for about 5 to 10 minutes before cutting into it. Resting doesn't magically lock in every drop of juice, but it does help the juices settle back into the meat. If you cut too early, more of that moisture ends up on the cutting board instead of in your mouth.

The reverse sear works especially well for ribeyes, strip steaks, thick pork chops, large lamb chops, and roasts you want to finish with a crust. It takes longer than a basic pan sear, but it's far more forgiving and usually produces a better result.

Technique B: The Cold Sear

The cold sear is one of the most underrated ways to cook fatty meats. It works especially well with bacon, duck breast, pork belly, and other cuts where the goal isn't just to cook the meat but to slowly melt and crisp the fat. Instead of starting with a hot pan, you place the meat in a cold pan and let the heat rise gradually.

This matters because fat needs time to render. Render just means the fat slowly melts out of the meat. If you throw fatty meat into a screaming hot pan too soon, the outside can burn before the fat underneath has time to melt properly. Starting cold and slowly bringing the pan up to medium or medium-low heat gives the fat time to soften, release, and brown evenly. The result is better texture, more usable cooking fat, and less risk of burning the outside while the inside stays chewy or undercooked.

For duck breast, this method is especially useful. Lightly scoring the skin before placing it skin-side down in a cold pan helps the fat melt out and lets the skin crisp as the pan heats up. For bacon, the cold sear reduces curling, cooks the strips more evenly, and gives you better control over how crispy you want the final result.

COOKING FROM FROZEN

Life happens. Meat doesn't always get thawed on time. That doesn't mean the plan has to fall apart. It doesn't mean you need to grab a cheat meal, order fast food, or tell yourself you'll start again tomorrow. One of the most practical skills in a carnivore kitchen is learning how to cook meat from frozen without ruining it. This isn't about making the perfect meal. It's about having a backup plan that keeps you consistent when the day doesn't go perfectly.

The air fryer is one of the best tools for this. Frozen burger patties, sausages, wings, and even smaller steaks can cook surprisingly well when they have enough hot air moving around them. Frozen burger patties usually do well at 400°F for about 12 to 15 minutes, flipped halfway through, depending on how thick they are. Use a meat thermometer when needed, especially with ground beef, because ground meat may need to be cooked all the way through. Depending on your preferences. The result may not be exactly the same as fresh meat, but it's good enough to keep you on plan, and that matters more on busy days. I've found that one-inch-thick frozen ribeyes or New York strips can cook well in about 18 to 20 minutes, flipped halfway through, for a medium-rare to medium result. You'll need to practice, because cooking times can vary depending on the air fryer, the thickness of the meat, and how frozen the meat is.

The slow cooker is another useful backup option, but this is where food safety matters. Large frozen roasts or big frozen blocks of ground meat shouldn't be placed directly into a slow cooker because they may stay in the unsafe temperature range too long before they fully heat through. A slow cooker works best when the meat is thawed or at least partially thawed. This is especially useful for chuck roast, stew meat, brisket, oxtail, short ribs, or other tougher cuts that benefit from long, slow cooking. Slow-cooked meat won't have the same texture as seared meat, but it's still nourishing, practical, and a lot better than falling back into processed food.

Avoiding the Common Mistakes

Most beginners make the same basic cooking mistakes. They crowd too much meat into the pan, which traps steam and prevents browning. They flip the meat too often, which keeps a good crust from forming. They try to sear meat while the surface is still wet, which almost guarantees a weak crust. They're afraid of salt, skip the resting period, or guess when the meat is done instead of checking the internal temperature.

These mistakes aren't complicated, but they add up. They're enough to turn good meat into boring, dry, gray food. When that happens repeatedly, carnivore starts to feel harder than it needs to be.

The fix is simple. Dry the surface of the meat before cooking. Use enough salt. Let the pan get hot before the meat goes in. Don't crowd the pan. Use a thermometer when needed. Let the meat rest before cutting into it. Most importantly, match the cooking method to the cut of meat. A ribeye, a chuck roast, ground beef, liver, and pork belly don't all need the same treatment. Choose the right method for the cut, and the meal will turn out better.

Batch Cooking Without Burnout: Meal Prep

Cooking skill isn't just about making one perfect steak. It's also about making this lifestyle easier across the whole week. Batch cooking can keep you from having to start from scratch every time you're hungry. You can cook several burger patties at once, brown a few pounds of ground beef, slow-cook a roast for multiple meals, or render extra tallow while cooking. All of that reduces future effort.

This matters because life gets busy. Hunger plus an empty kitchen is a bad combination. A person with cooked meat in the refrigerator has a much better shot at staying on plan than a person standing hungry with nothing ready. Meal prep helps remove frustration. It makes the right choice easier before you're tired, stressed, or tempted.

Bottom Line

If you want carnivore to work long-term, your food must be worth eating. Technique is what makes that possible. You don't need to become a chef, but you do need to learn a few reliable methods. Understand heat. Use salt.

Learn when to sear, when to slow cook, when to air fry, and when to let the meat rest.

Stop treating meat like a plain slab of protein that can be cooked any random way. Meat responds to how you handle it. When you choose the right method for the cut and cook it well, the food becomes more satisfying. And when the food is satisfying, the lifestyle becomes a whole lot easier to maintain.

BUDGET CARNIVORE

One of the biggest myths about carnivore is that it's only possible for people with a lot of money to spend on food. That's false. Carnivore can get expensive if you insist on ribeye every night, fancy supplements, branded "keto" snacks, and convenience foods pretending to be health products. But that isn't the only way to do it. In many cases, people may actually spend less when they stop buying snacks, soft drinks, desserts, sauces, side dishes, and restaurant meals made with cheap ingredients but sold at high prices.

A budget carnivore approach works when you stop thinking like a modern shopper chasing labels and start thinking like someone trying to get the most nutrition for the money. That means focusing on nutrient-dense staples, buying in bulk when possible, choosing cuts based on value instead of status, and not wasting the fat and juices that come with the meat.

THE GROUND BEEF STRATEGY

Ground beef is the backbone of budget carnivore. It's easy to find, easy to cook, easy to store, easy to prepare in batches, and one of the most cost-effective ways to build your diet around ruminant meat.

Fattier blends like 70/30 or 80/20 are usually the better choice for this approach. The fat does more than add flavor, it adds fullness and energy, which helps the meal last longer and keeps you from needing more food soon after. Lean ground beef may look "cleaner" to someone still thinking in low-fat diet terms, but it can be a false bargain. If you buy lean meat and then feel hungry an hour later because the meal didn't satisfy you, you didn't really save money. You just pushed the cost to later.

When you cook ground beef, don't automatically drain the fat. In a carnivore framework, the rendered fat isn't trash. It's part of the food you paid for, and it's part of the energy that makes the meal work. Pouring it off and then wondering why you're hungry soon after is a classic beginner mistake. If the fat is too much for your digestion at first, ease into it. But don't throw it away just because old low-fat habits told you to.

INEXPENSIVE GEMS

Some of the best foods in a budget carnivore plan are the cuts modern people overlook because they take more time to cook. Chuck roast, brisket, beef shanks, short ribs, stew meat, oxtail, and pork shoulder are good examples. These cuts often cost less than premium steaks, but they can still give you a lot of flavor, fat, and satisfaction when they're cooked properly.

These cuts are usually tougher because they contain more connective tissue and collagen. That doesn't make them bad, it just means they need the right cooking method. Slow cooking, pressure cooking, braising, or cooking low and slow in the oven can turn tough cuts into tender, rich, satisfying meals. Once you learn how to cook them, these cheaper cuts may become some of your favorite foods in the entire diet.

This is where patience becomes part of your budget strategy. The grocery store charges more for tenderness and convenience. If you're willing to use a slow cooker, an Instant Pot, or a low oven for a few hours, you can often eat very well for much less money.

Eggs can also be useful if you tolerate them well. They're usually affordable, easy to cook, and packed with useful nutrients, protein, choline, vitamin A. They're not the foundation of carnivore the way ruminant meat is, but they help stretch meals, add convenience, and give you variety without wrecking your grocery budget.

Buying Smarter, Not Fancier

One of the easiest ways to lower cost is to shop by price per pound instead of by brand image. Family packs, manager's specials, bulk ground beef, freezer sales, and larger cuts of meat can all save money if you have the freezer space and are willing to portion the meat yourself. A chest freezer isn't exciting, but for someone eating animal foods regularly, it can become one of the best money-saving tools in the house.

It also helps to think in terms of meal value instead of food status. A ribeye may feel premium, but several pounds of ground beef, a chuck roast, or a pork shoulder may give you more total meals, more fullness, and less financial stress. The goal isn't to impress anyone with your grocery cart. The goal is to stay fed, stay consistent, and get the most nourishment you can for the money.

What to Avoid on a Budget

The fastest way to make carnivore more expensive than it needs to be is to buy products marketed to people who don't know better. "Keto" bars, carnivore-branded snacks, flavored electrolyte drinks, protein chips, expensive jerky, and designer convenience products are usually overpriced, less filling, and less nutritious than plain meat. They aren't helping you save money. Most of the time, they're processed snack foods wearing a health label.

The same logic applies to many processed deli meats and convenience foods. These products often contain added sugars, fillers, preservatives, and other ingredients you don't need. You may see ingredients like dextrose, carrageenan, starches, gums, or flavoring agents. That doesn't mean every slice of deli meat is poison, and it doesn't mean you can never use convenience foods in a pinch. But if you're trying to build a clean, affordable carnivore diet, whole cuts of meat, ground beef, eggs if tolerated, and slow-cooked cheaper roasts usually give you better value and fewer unnecessary ingredients.

On a budget, simplicity wins twice. It's usually cheaper, and it gives the body fewer extra ingredients to deal with.

THE QUALITY QUESTION

Budget carnivore doesn't mean food quality doesn't matter. Better sourcing is still better when you can afford it. But you need to keep the order straight. First, eat animal foods consistently. Second, make ruminant meat, beef, lamb, bison, deer, and elk, the foundation. Third, improve sourcing when your budget allows.

Don't let perfect sourcing become an excuse to keep eating junk. The jump from processed food to regular grocery store beef is much bigger than the jump from regular beef to premium grass-finished beef. If all you can afford right now is conventional ground beef, start there. That's still a major upgrade from cereal, chips, fast food, frozen meals, and snack foods.

SUMMARY OF CHAPTER 3

Chapter 3 turned theory into action. Up to this point, the carnivore framework has been built on biology, food quality, and nutrition logic. In this chapter, the focus shifted to real life, how to set up your kitchen, how to cook meat well enough to enjoy it, and how to make this way of eating work without needing an unlimited grocery budget.

The main lesson is simple: success on carnivore isn't built on motivation alone. Motivation fades. Systems last longer. If your kitchen is set up well, your food tastes good, your meals are easy to repeat, and your freezer has meat ready to go, you're much more likely to stay consistent. The easier you make the right choice, the more often you'll make it.

We started with the carnivore toolkit. Long-term success doesn't require a luxury kitchen or a pile of expensive gadgets. It requires a few practical tools that make cooking easier and more consistent. A cast iron skillet, a sharp knife, a large cutting board, a digital meat thermometer, and basic storage containers create the foundation. Optional tools like an air fryer, sous vide cooker, slow cooker, Instant Pot, and freezer can make the process even easier, especially if you cook in bulk or use cheaper cuts of meat. The point isn't to look like a chef. The point is to make meat easier to cook, store, and enjoy.

From there, we moved into cooking mastery. A lot of people don't fail on carnivore because meat doesn't work for them, they fail because they never learn to cook it properly. Dry, overcooked, boring meals eventually wear people down. By learning techniques like the reverse sear, cold sear, cooking from frozen, slow cooking, and batch cooking, you give yourself more ways to make meat satisfying. You also learn how to match the right method to the right cut instead of treating every piece of meat the same way.

You also saw that carnivore doesn't require premium steaks, expensive products, or an elite grocery budget. It requires priorities. Ground beef is one of the best budget tools because it's affordable, easy to cook, easy to store, and filling when you choose fattier blends. Cheaper cuts like chuck roast, brisket, stew meat, beef shanks, short ribs, and pork shoulder aren't inferior foods, they just need better cooking methods. When cooked properly, they can become some of the most satisfying meals in the entire diet.

Eggs, if tolerated, can also play a useful supporting role because they're affordable, easy to prepare, and nutrient dense. The chapter also made clear what not to waste money on, processed "keto" products, designer convenience foods, expensive snack replacements, and heavily marketed products that add cost without adding real nourishment.

The lesson is blunt: budget carnivore works when you spend your money on actual food and stop spending it on things pretending to be food.

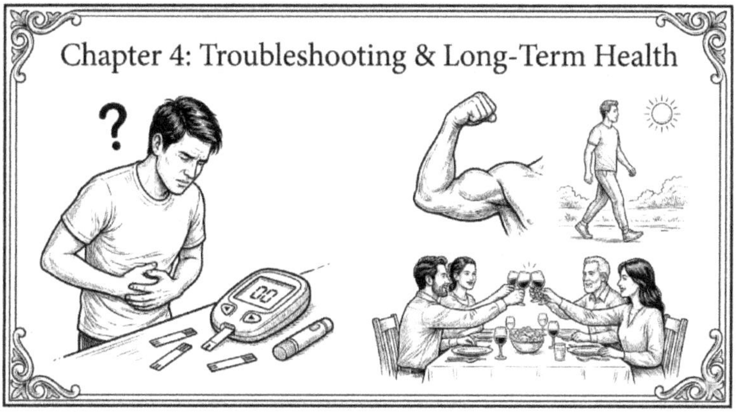
Chapter 4: Troubleshooting & Long-Term Health
?

CHAPTER 4

TROUBLESHOOTING & LONG-TERM HEALTH

One of the most common mistakes people make on carnivore is assuming that if the diet makes sense, the body should respond immediately, smoothly, and without any problems. That isn't how adaptation works. A body that has spent years dealing with processed food, chronic stress, unstable hunger signals, poor sleep, blood sugar swings, and inconsistent recovery doesn't suddenly become steady overnight. It changes in stages. Those stages can sometimes feel uncomfortable, confusing, or easy to misread.

Digestion may change before it stabilizes. Bloodwork may improve in some areas while raising questions in others. Morning blood sugar may rise in a way that seems backward until you understand what's happening hormonally. Women may discover that eating enough matters more than proving how strict they can be. Training performance may dip before the body fully adapts to using fat as fuel. Sleep may feel lighter or more broken before it gets deeper and more stable. Social situations may become more difficult, not because the diet is wrong, but because the people around you don't always understand your consistency. None of these experiences automatically means something is wrong. But none of them should be ignored either. The real skill is learning the difference between normal adaptation, poor execution, and problems that deserve closer attention.

This chapter is designed to teach that skill. It'll help you understand digestive changes without panic, look at bloodwork with more nuance, see how hormones and performance can shift under a new fuel system, and handle social pressure without giving up your standards. The goal isn't to promise a perfect transition or pretend every symptom is harmless. The goal is to give you a framework for responding intelligently.

Digestion Troubleshooting: The Gut's Great Migration

The digestive tract is usually the first place people notice changes when they transition to carnivore. That isn't surprising. For years, sometimes decades, the gut has been operating under one set of inputs: plant matter, fiber, starch, sugar, mixed meals, additives, and frequent eating. When that environment changes suddenly, digestion changes with it. Stool volume changes. Bowel frequency changes. Gas patterns change. Fat tolerance changes. In that sense, the gut isn't necessarily failing. It's adapting.

Part of that adaptation likely involves the microbiome, but this is an area worth discussing carefully. The gut microbiome responds to diet, and ketogenic or very low-carbohydrate diets can change microbial patterns and gut-related signals. But the exact changes are complex and not fully settled. The practical point is simpler: when you remove most fermentable plant material and shift toward a meat-and-fat-based diet, the digestive environment changes quickly. Some digestive symptoms during that adjustment are common.

- **Issue A: The Challenge of "Disaster Pants" (Diarrhea)**

Loose stools early in carnivore are common enough that they deserve a direct discussion. In many cases, the problem isn't infection, food poisoning, or proof that the diet is wrong. It's often a mismatch between fat intake, bile handling, meal size, and digestive adaptation.

One useful way to think about this is overload. Rendered liquid fat is usually harder for beginners to handle than fat that's naturally attached to the meat. If a large amount of fat reaches the intestine in a form your body doesn't handle well yet, urgency and loose stools can follow. In medical terms, bile acids reaching the colon are known to contribute to loose stool, urgency, and frequent bowel movements in a condition called bile acid diarrhea. That doesn't mean every loose stool episode on carnivore is officially bile acid diarrhea. It simply means the basic idea makes sense: eating more fat increases bile activity in the gut, and too much bile reaching the colon can create diarrhea-like symptoms.

This is where the form of the fat matters. Many people tolerate the natural fat in a ribeye, chuck roast, or ground beef better than a cup of pan drippings, melted butter, or straight liquid tallow poured on top. This is me. Liquid fat goes right through me. A useful rule during early adaptation is simple, don't drink your fat. If loose stools are a problem, reduce rendered liquid fat for a while, keep eating fatty meat, and give your digestive system time to adjust. Choose solid animal fat that comes with the meat instead of pouring extra grease over everything.

If symptoms are mild, the fix is often simple. Reduce free liquid fat temporarily. Split very large meals into smaller meals. Keep sodium and hydration in a reasonable range. Favor fatty whole cuts over drinking or pouring large amounts of grease onto the plate. For many people, this settles as adaptation improves. But if diarrhea is persistent, severe, or comes with weight loss, nighttime urgency, fever, blood, or significant abdominal pain, don't treat that as normal transition. That needs medical evaluation.

- **Issue B: Constipation or Just Low Residue?**

The other common fear is the opposite problem: "I'm not going every day, so something must be wrong." Sometimes that concern is valid. Often, it isn't.

A lower-residue diet naturally produces less stool. If most of what you eat is being digested and absorbed, there's simply less waste left over to eliminate. Less output doesn't automatically mean constipation.

True constipation usually means difficult passage, straining, pain, bloating, or a feeling that you still need to go but can't fully empty. A bowel movement every two or three days, without discomfort, may simply mean your body is producing less stool. This is one reason people new to carnivore often mistake normal adaptation for a problem. The system is producing less waste, so the pattern changes.

Fiber makes this discussion more complicated because the evidence isn't one-size-fits-all. The honest answer isn't "fiber is always good" or "fiber is always bad." The honest answer is that bowel function depends on context. Eating less fiber doesn't automatically mean you'll become constipated.

When true constipation does happen on carnivore, the usual causes are practical. Too little fluid for your needs. Too little sodium. Too little total food. In some cases, too little fat. Sometimes the digestive system is simply still adapting to a very different way of eating. That's why the first response should be supportive, not panicked. Increase fluids sensibly. Make sure sodium intake is adequate. Make sure the diet hasn't accidentally turned into lean protein because you're still afraid of fat. Some people also find magnesium helpful for short-term relief, especially magnesium citrate, because it can pull water into the bowel.

THE BROADER PRINCIPLE

The larger lesson in digestion troubleshooting is that early changes don't always mean damage. Often, they mean adaptation. The digestive system is responding to different foods, a different meal pattern, and a different hormonal environment. Some of that adjustment may feel smooth. Some of it may feel awkward. The mistake is assuming every change from your old normal is automatically a sign that something is wrong.

If stools are loose, look first at rendered liquid fat, meal size, and time. If stool frequency drops, ask whether there's true discomfort or simply less waste being produced. If symptoms are severe or persistent, don't romanticize them. Use judgment and get medical help when needed. But don't sabotage the process by treating every temporary digestive shift as proof that the diet is broken.

The most useful mindset is this: interpret before you react. The gut isn't always speaking the language of emergency. Sometimes it's simply speaking the language of change.

Bloodwork: Interpreting the New Metadata

If you get bloodwork during the first few months of carnivore, you may find yourself in a confusing conversation. On one hand, triglycerides may fall, HDL may rise, fasting glucose may improve, and many people feel metabolically steadier. On the other hand, LDL cholesterol may rise, sometimes dramatically. That combination can unsettle both patients and physicians, especially when the conversation treats every cholesterol marker the same way in every person. The truth is more complicated. Low-carbohydrate eating can change the way energy is stored, transported, and used, but that doesn't mean traditional cardiovascular risk markers suddenly stop mattering. It means they need to be interpreted carefully.

This is where many people make one of two mistakes. Some panic the moment LDL rises and assume the diet is damaging them. Others dismiss any LDL increase as automatically harmless because triglycerides are low and HDL is high. The stronger position is this, carbohydrate restriction can produce a distinct lipid pattern in some people, especially leaner people with low triglycerides and high HDL, but the long-term meaning of very high LDL in that context is still being debated and studied. It isn't a closed case.

THE LEAN MASS HYPER-RESPONDER (LMHR)

One pattern that has drawn more attention is called the Lean Mass Hyper-Responder, or LMHR. This term is used to describe people, often lean, insulin-sensitive, and eating a carbohydrate-restricted diet, who develop very high LDL cholesterol along with low triglycerides and high HDL.

This pattern appears to be real in the sense that it has been observed and described in published research. What remains unresolved is what it means for long-term risk. One popular explanation is that in a fat-adapted state, LDL particles may reflect increased energy transport, with VLDL and LDL helping move triglycerides and cholesterol to tissues. That idea is biologically plausible and may help explain why some lean people see large LDL changes when carbohydrate intake falls and fat becomes the main fuel source.

A 2024 study looked at LMHR and near-LMHR individuals on carbohydrate-restricted diets with LDL-C of at least 190 mg/dL and compared their coronary plaque burden with matched controls. The study reported that baseline LDL-C wasn't associated with baseline coronary plaque burden in that cohort. That's important, but it isn't the same as proving long-term safety. It was a specific study in a specific group, and longer-term outcomes still matter.

That's the mature position: LMHR appears to be a legitimate phenotype, and carbohydrate restriction can markedly increase LDL in some lean, metabolically healthy people. But there isn't enough evidence yet to claim that high LDL in this context is automatically harmless. A 2026 review described the clinical meaning of LDL elevation in LMHRs as an unresolved question and noted that it doesn't erase the broader established role of LDL-C in atherosclerotic cardiovascular disease.

A useful resource for understanding this debate is Dave Feldman's work on Lean Mass Hyper-Responders and the documentary "The Cholesterol Code". The film was released in 2026 and follows Feldman's work around ketogenic diets, LDL cholesterol, and the LMHR phenotype. I'm not associated with Feldman or the documentary, and this shouldn't be treated as medical advice. But if you're going to discuss cholesterol seriously in the low-carb or carnivore space, this is one of the conversations worth understanding.

The Numbers That Matter

This is why a single number rarely tells the whole story. Total cholesterol by itself is often a blunt and limited marker. It combines several different things into one large number, which can create more anxiety than clarity. A better first step is to look at the overall pattern.

Triglycerides matter because they can give you clues about carbohydrate intake, insulin resistance, and how the body is handling energy. On lower-carbohydrate diets, triglycerides often decrease. HDL often rises as well. That pattern is usually viewed as a favorable sign, but it still needs to be interpreted alongside the rest of the picture.

That's why the triglyceride-to-HDL ratio can be useful. It's often used as a simple marker that may reflect insulin sensitivity and metabolic health. A lower TG/HDL ratio is generally associated with better insulin sensitivity and lower cardiometabolic risk, while a higher ratio often tracks with metabolic syndrome and insulin resistance. That said, it's still a proxy marker. It can be useful, but it isn't a perfect diagnostic tool, and cutoffs may vary between individuals and populations.

In practical terms, many people view triglycerides below 100 mg/dL as encouraging, especially when paired with good glucose control, lower waist circumference, and improving body composition. HDL that's rising or strong is also generally viewed favorably. A TG/HDL ratio around 1.0 or lower is often considered a strong metabolic signal, but it isn't a magic number. It tells you something useful about insulin sensitivity and energy handling. It doesn't erase every other risk marker.

What to Do With a Rising LDL

If LDL rises modestly while triglycerides improve, HDL improves, body composition improves, blood pressure improves, and other metabolic markers move in the right direction, that conversation is different from a situation where LDL rises into very high ranges while the rest of the metabolic picture looks poor. Context matters.

Extreme LDL elevations deserve attention. This is especially true if LDL is very high while HDL is low, triglycerides are high, blood pressure is elevated, blood sugar is poor, waist circumference is high, or there's a strong family history of early heart disease. That isn't a situation to ignore or explain away with diet ideology.

That's why I wouldn't frame bloodwork on carnivore as "ignore LDL." A better frame is, interpret the whole pattern, and increase the level of scrutiny when the numbers call for it. Total cholesterol is crude. Triglycerides and HDL can tell you a lot about metabolic state. But non-HDL cholesterol, and when appropriate, imaging such as coronary artery calcium scoring or coronary CT angiography may provide a more complete picture than arguing endlessly over LDL by itself. Recent cholesterol guidance continues to emphasize LDL-C and non-HDL-C goals, while imaging can help refine risk in the right context.

THE PRACTICAL LESSON

The most useful lesson here isn't to become dismissive of bloodwork, but to become more literate in it. Carnivore can improve some markers quickly while complicating others. That means you need context, not panic. Low triglycerides and high HDL are generally favorable signs. Total cholesterol alone tells you little. Marked LDL elevation on carbohydrate restriction may reflect a real metabolic response in certain people, especially leaner individuals, but the long-term consequences are still not fully settled.

So, when you look at labs, don't ask only, did LDL go up? Ask better questions. What happened to my triglycerides? What happened to my HDL? What's my TG/HDL ratio? What's my non-HDL cholesterol? What's my apoB if it was tested? What's my family history? What's happening with my blood pressure, waist circumference, glucose control, fasting insulin, inflammatory markers, and body composition? And if the LDL rise is large, what do repeat testing and deeper evaluation show over time?

On carnivore, bloodwork may change in ways that are metabolically favorable, clinically concerning, or both. Your job isn't to worship one number or dismiss another. Your job is to understand the pattern well enough to act intelligently.

BLOOD SUGAR & THE DAWN PHENOMENON

It can feel strange to wake up after a full night without eating, check your blood sugar, and see that it's higher than it was before bed. For many people, that feels backward. If you haven't eaten for ten or twelve hours, why would blood sugar go up instead of down? The answer is simple; the body isn't just sitting there waiting for food. It's always working. It regulates fuel based on time of day, hormones, sleep, stress, and what it expects you to need. One example of this is called the dawn phenomenon.

The dawn phenomenon is an early-morning rise in blood sugar that happens without food. It's most often discussed in diabetes research, but the basic idea applies more broadly. In the early-morning hours, hormones help prepare the body to wake up, move, and function. Hormones such as cortisol and growth hormone can signal the liver to release glucose into the bloodstream. In plain language, your body may raise blood sugar in the morning because it's preparing you for the day.

In practical terms, a slightly higher fasting glucose first thing in the morning doesn't automatically mean something is wrong. It may simply mean the body is doing what it's supposed to do, making a little fuel available so you can wake up and get moving. On carnivore or any very low-carbohydrate way of eating, this can become more noticeable because you're no longer constantly adding carbohydrates throughout the day.

This is where context matters. A fasting glucose of 100 mg/dL when you first wake up that comes down after eating, hydrating, or moving is a very different situation from fasting glucose that stays high, rises over time, comes with poor post-meal blood sugar control, or shows up alongside a rising A1c. The first may simply reflect normal morning hormone activity. The second deserves more attention. Blood sugar should be judged by patterns, not panic over one reading. A single number tells you far less than repeated readings viewed alongside A1c, fasting insulin when available, triglycerides, HDL, waist size, body composition, sleep, stress, and the rest of your health picture.

There's a practical lesson here. If your fasting glucose is mildly elevated in the morning but improves after food, water, or movement, don't immediately assume you're metabolically broken. Morning exercise can sometimes raise glucose temporarily too, especially if the dawn phenomenon is already happening. That's because exercise and morning hormones both increase the body's demand for fuel. That doesn't automatically mean failure. Often, it simply means the body is releasing fuel on schedule.

At the same time, this shouldn't become an excuse to explain away every abnormal reading. If fasting glucose is consistently high, if it keeps rising over time, if post-meal glucose control is poor, or if A1c is moving upward, that deserves attention from a qualified healthcare professional.

It's also a reason to look honestly at sleep, stress, total food intake, movement, meal timing, and whether the diet is being followed in a way that supports metabolic health.

The most useful interpretation is this: the dawn phenomenon reminds you that blood sugar is controlled by more than food alone. What you eat matters, but so do circadian rhythm, sleep, stress, liver output, hormones, and timing. On a carnivore diet, those patterns can sometimes become easier to see because the system is less cluttered.

A morning rise in glucose isn't always a sign of dysfunction. Sometimes it's simply the body announcing that the day has begun.

WOMEN'S HEALTH

Women's bodies aren't fragile, but they are very responsive to signals about energy, stress, and safety. That isn't a weakness, that's how the body is designed. Reproductive function takes a lot of energy, so the female body pays close attention to whether conditions are good enough to support ovulation, pregnancy, and long-term hormone balance. When food intake is too low, stress is too high, or the body senses ongoing scarcity, the menstrual cycle can start to change.

That's why women often need to be careful when combining low-carb eating, under-eating, hard training, and aggressive fasting. One of these by itself may be fine in the right situation. But when they're all stacked together, they can become a problem. The better way to say this isn't that women are "too sensitive." The better way to say it is that the female hormonal system is closely connected to energy, stress, and recovery. When the body senses that conditions aren't supportive, reproductive hormones are often one of the first systems to show the strain.

Because estrogen and progesterone are made from cholesterol, fat and cholesterol aren't enemies of female hormone health. They're part of the raw material the body uses to make these hormones. That doesn't mean simply eating more cholesterol will automatically fix hormone problems. Hormones are affected by the brain, ovaries, thyroid, adrenal system, sleep, stress, and overall food intake. But it does mean that a low-fat, underfed, high-stress lifestyle is a poor foundation for strong hormone health.

Warning Signs the System May Be Underfed

When a woman starts under-recovering on a restrictive or poorly planned diet, the body often gives warning signs before a formal medical problem is diagnosed. Hair thinning, feeling cold easily, low sex drive, poor recovery, sleep problems, mood swings, and irregular cycles can all be signs that the body is under too much strain or not getting enough energy. None of these symptoms is unique to carnivore, and none should be blamed on one thing automatically. But they shouldn't be ignored either. Menstrual cycle changes are one of the clearest signs that the body may not be getting enough support, and symptoms like cold intolerance and hair changes can also point to broader stress on the system.

The practical lesson is simple, don't treat these warning signs as proof that you need more discipline. In many cases, they're signs that you need more support. A woman who's training hard, fasting aggressively, and eating too little may not need more restriction. She may need more food, more recovery, more sleep, and a less combative approach to the diet. This is especially true if the goal is long-term health instead of short-term weight-loss theater.

THE SOLUTION: FUEL FIRST, STRESS SECOND

In practical terms, the first correction is usually making sure total food intake is high enough. That often means eating more, not obsessing over perfect macros. On a carnivore approach, this may mean more total calories, more fat, and less accidental under-eating. If meals are too lean, portions are too small, or fasting windows are too aggressive, the body may read the whole situation as scarcity.

The second correction is often reducing how often extended fasting is used, especially if cycle changes, hair thinning, or feeling cold all the time are showing up. Fasting can be useful in some situations, but it isn't a moral achievement. Women don't always respond to aggressive fasting the same way men do. If the body is already stressed, adding more stress rarely helps. A better strategy is often to stabilize meals, eat until satisfied, protect sleep as a non-negotiable recovery tool, and allow the body's hormonal rhythm to steady before experimenting with stricter fasting windows again.

THE MATURE VIEW

The mature view of women's hormones on carnivore isn't ideological. It's adaptive. Some women do very well on a strict carnivore approach. Others do better with more total food, more dietary fat, less fasting, less training stress, or a more flexible approach depending on symptoms, cycle status, and goals. The female body gives feedback all the time. The job isn't to ignore that feedback in order to defend a diet identity. The job is to listen to it and adjust.

For women, hormonal health is rarely improved by proving how little you can survive on. It improves when the body receives a clear signal that food is sufficient, stress is manageable, and the environment is stable enough for normal reproductive function to continue.

EXERCISE PERFORMANCE

Don't expect your best gym performance during the first few weeks of carnivore. For many people, there's an adjustment period. The body is changing how it uses fuel, shifting water and electrolyte balance, changing how it stores and uses glycogen, and learning to rely more on fat for energy. During that transition, performance may feel different before it feels better. You may feel flat, less explosive, less springy, and more aware of effort during workouts that normally feel routine.

This is often a sign that the body is still adapting, not proof that the diet is failing. Research on ketogenic and very low-carbohydrate diets shows that the body can increase fat burning, but performance results are mixed. Strength is often maintained better than high-intensity performance, while sprinting, intervals, and repeated hard efforts are more likely to suffer, especially early in the transition.

This matters most for people whose training depends on quick, explosive energy. That includes sprinting, repeated intervals, CrossFit-style workouts, hard sparring, explosive lifting, and any training where speed and power matter. Those systems don't disappear on carnivore, but they may feel less available while the body adapts. Endurance at moderate effort may hold steady for some people, but high-intensity work is often where the drop shows up first.

That's why the phrase adaptive dip is more useful than calling it failure. Your body isn't necessarily becoming weaker in every way. It's changing fuel systems, and that takes time. In the first two to three weeks, many people notice less explosiveness, heavier legs, slower recovery between hard efforts, and a feeling that the nervous system isn't firing as sharply. Some of this may come from glycogen changes. Some may come from water and sodium shifts. Some is simply the body learning how to perform under a different fuel setup.

That doesn't mean every type of performance drops the same way. Maximal strength often holds up better than repeated high-intensity output. In practical terms, you may still be able to lift heavy weight reasonably well, but bar speed, repeated sprints, hard conditioning, and explosive efforts may feel worse at first.

Endurance is more nuanced. Some people report steadier long-duration energy and less need for constant fueling once they adapt. The body can become better at using fat for energy. But that doesn't automatically mean endurance performance will improve. In some trained athletes, using more fat for fuel may come with a tradeoff, the body may need more oxygen to hold the same pace, especially at higher intensities. The mature message isn't that endurance will definitely get better. The mature message is that some people may feel more stable during long efforts, but performance benefits aren't guaranteed. It depends on the sport, the intensity, the athlete, and how long adaptation takes.

What should you do during this phase? First, lower your expectations temporarily without lowering your standards. This isn't the time to judge the diet by whether you can hit a personal record in week two. Keep training but consider reducing volume or intensity slightly until the body settles. Use this period to maintain movement quality, technique, and consistency instead of chasing peak output while your system is still adapting.

Second, support the body while it adapts. Sodium and hydration matter. When carbohydrates drop very low, the body often loses more water and sodium, especially in the beginning. That can affect blood volume, muscle contraction, energy, and how hard exercise feels. Adding salt to pre-workout water can be a useful step for many people. The bigger point is simple, during the transition, don't ignore salt and fluids. They can make a major difference.

Adequate food intake matters too. A person trying to adapt to carnivore while under-eating, fearing fat, and training hard is stacking stress on top of stress. That's a poor setup. If you want your body to perform, you have to give it enough fuel to work with.

Third, be honest about the difference between adaptation and identity. If your sport, job, or livelihood depends on maximum performance, you need to be honest about tradeoffs. Carnivore may improve appetite control, body composition, metabolic stability, and day-to-day energy for some people, but that doesn't automatically make it the best setup for every athletic goal. A more disciplined conclusion is this, carnivore may work well in some situations, may be neutral in others, and may hurt certain types of high-intensity performance.

The practical rule is simple. In the first few weeks, expect a dip. Don't panic. Support electrolytes. Eat enough food. Train intelligently. Give the body time to adapt before making final judgments. If performance later stabilizes and you feel strong, steady, and recovered, that's useful feedback. If your specific sport continues to suffer after a meaningful adaptation period, that's useful feedback too.

Social Situations & Dining Out

For most people, the hardest part of carnivore isn't hunger, cravings, or even cooking. It's social pressure. Modern life is built around shared food. Birthdays, business meetings, holidays, date nights, family gatherings, and casual lunches all usually involve foods that people expect everyone to eat without question. The moment you stop following that expectation, you're not just making a food choice, you're breaking the usual script. That's why social pressure knocks so many people off track. The real challenge isn't the steak on your plate. The challenge is often the discomfort other people feel when your discipline makes them notice their own habits.

If you wait until the food arrives and everyone is watching, you're already in a weaker position. Carnivore becomes much easier when you decide ahead of time what you'll order, how you'll respond, and what you'll say if someone questions you. The goal isn't to convert anyone, defend your diet in public, or win an argument over dinner. The goal is to protect your standard without turning every meal into a debate.

THE SCRIPT: CALM, SIMPLE, FINAL

Most social pressure works because people sense uncertainty. If you sound unsure, apologetic, or open to negotiation, people will push. If you sound calm and matter of fact, most people will move on. That's why your response should be simple, polite, and final.

A useful script: "I'm on a strict elimination diet right now to troubleshoot some issues."

That line works because it's simple, true enough, and not dramatic. It signals that this isn't a fad, not a casual preference, and not an invitation for argument. Most people will respect a health-based boundary more than a diet debate. They may not understand carnivore, but they understand the idea of trying to figure out what foods work for your body.

Other strong variations:

"I'm keeping food very simple right now."

"I'm testing what I tolerate, so I'm staying strict."

"I feel better when I eat this way, so I'm sticking with it."

The exact words matter less than the tone. Calm. Brief. No apology. No lecture.

What Not to Do

Don't over-explain. The more you explain, the more openings you create for people to challenge you. Don't start talking about insulin, lectins, seed oils, or human evolution unless someone sincerely asks in private and you actually want to have that conversation. Most public food pressure isn't intellectual, it's social. Long explanations don't end social pressure. They usually feed it.

Don't describe your choice like it's a temporary weakness. Phrases like "I'm trying to be good" or "I'm not supposed to" make your decision sound fragile. Say what you're doing, not what you're trying to resist.

And don't expect approval. You don't need it. The goal isn't for everyone to understand. The goal is to leave the meal knowing you kept your standard.

Restaurant Strategy: Make the Environment Work for You

Dining out doesn't have to destroy the diet, but it does require better decision-making. Restaurants are built to sell combinations, bread with meat, fries with burgers, chips with salsa, dessert with drinks. Your job is to strip the meal down to the parts that actually serve you.

- ***Steakhouses***

This is usually the easiest environment. Order a ribeye, New York strip, sirloin, burger patty, or another plain cut of meat. Ask for butter if you tolerate dairy. Skip the sides, or substitute extra meat, eggs, or plain burger patties when available. Salt the food generously and keep the order simple.

- ***Burger Joints***

Burger places are very workable if you ignore the packaging. Order multiple patties with no bun, no sauce, and no sugary condiments. Cheese is optional if you tolerate dairy. Bacon can work if the ingredients are clean enough and you do well with pork. In most cases, three or four patties are far more useful than a burger meal built around fries and soda.

- ***Mexican Restaurants***

Mexican restaurants require more precision because almost everything comes wrapped, topped, or mixed with something else. Fajita meat, grilled steak, carnitas, or plain ground beef can work well if you can get them without tortillas, beans, rice, chips, or sugary marinades. Ask for plain meat when possible. Ignore the chips on the table entirely. Once you start "just having a few," the standard is already breaking down.

- ***Breakfast Restaurants***

Breakfast spots are often underrated for carnivore. Eggs, bacon, sausage, burger patties, steak, hamburger steak, or omelets stripped down to meat and eggs can all work. Skip the toast, pancakes, hash browns, fruit cups, and syrups. Breakfast menus are often one of the easiest ways to eat simply in a social setting.

- ***Barbecue***

Barbecue can be excellent or terrible depending on how much sugar the restaurant uses in the rubs and sauces. Brisket, sliced beef, sausage, or pulled pork may work well, but sauces should usually be avoided unless you know what's in them. Dry meat is better than sugary meat disguised as barbecue.

- ***Buffets and Family Gatherings***

These settings reward scanning before serving. Look for the simplest animal foods first, carved meat, burger patties, roast beef, ham, turkey, deviled eggs, shrimp, or plain cheese if tolerated. Build the plate around what's clearly useful. Don't start with "just a little" of the fillers. Start with meat. Finish with meat. Make the rest irrelevant.

The Order Matters

One of the best tactics in social eating is ordering first when possible. If you order decisively, you set your standard before the social momentum builds. If you wait and listen to everyone else negotiate appetizers, desserts, cocktails, and side dishes, it becomes easier to drift. Decisive ordering protects discipline.

Another useful tactic is to eat beforehand if you know the event will be weak on good options. A person who arrives already fed is much harder to pressure than a person who arrives hungry and hopes the menu will cooperate.

- **Alcohol: The Social Trap**

Alcohol deserves special caution because it lowers judgment before it lowers anything else. Many people notice that when carbohydrates are lower and food is simpler, alcohol feels different. Even if your tolerance hasn't truly "collapsed," the combination of less glycogen, less food volume, and fewer blood sugar swings can make alcohol hit harder and feel less forgiving.

If you choose to drink, be strategic. Clear spirits with soda water or very dry wine are usually less disruptive than beer, sweet cocktails, margaritas, or sugary mixed drinks.

But the bigger point isn't which alcohol is "allowed." The bigger point is that alcohol is often the first crack in decision-making. One drink lowers standards. Two drinks usually lower them more. That's how a disciplined meal turns into a "weekend exception."

If the event matters more than the drinking, protect the event and skip the alcohol. Most people regret the compromise more than they enjoy the drink.

Remember this, when you drink, your body must deal with the alcohol first. Fat burning slows down. Blood sugar can become less stable. Sleep quality can suffer. Digestion can be irritated. Alcohol gives the body nothing useful while forcing it to work harder to clear it out.

- **The Deeper Problem: Food as Tribal Signaling**

Part of what makes social eating difficult is that food is rarely just food. When you refuse certain foods, some people may hear rejection, even when you don't mean it that way. That's why reactions can feel strangely emotional. You're not just declining cake. In their mind, you may be declining participation in the group ritual.

Understanding this helps you stay calm. You don't have to take every reaction personally. Often, the tension has more to do with what your choice represents to the other person than with what's actually on your plate. If you understand that, you can stay polite without becoming defensive.

The Long Game

No single meal determines success. But repeated compromise, especially when it's justified by social convenience, absolutely can. That's why your standard must be clear. If your default is strong, an occasional imperfect meal stays an exception. If your default is weak, every social event becomes a reset button.

The mature goal isn't isolation. It's controlled participation. You can go out. You can travel. You can celebrate. You can sit at the table without surrendering your standards. But that only happens when you stop treating every invitation like a surprise test and start treating it like something you already know how to handle.

Bottom Line

Social situations don't defeat carnivore. Lack of preparation does. Have your script. Know your order. Eat first if needed. Let other people have their discomfort if they need to. Your job isn't to make everyone comfortable with your choices. Your job is to make choices you can respect when the meal is over.

SUMMARY OF CHAPTER 4

In this chapter, we moved beyond the question of what to eat and into the more demanding task of understanding what your body is telling you once the diet is in motion. Carnivore doesn't always produce a perfectly smooth transition. Many of the changes people experience early on can be misread as failure when they're actually signals. The purpose of this chapter was to help you tell the difference between normal adaptation, poor execution, and situations that deserve closer attention. The central lesson is that long-term success depends less on panic or blind faith and more on disciplined interpretation.

We began with digestion, where the first signs of change often appear. Loose stools, urgency, and changes in bowel frequency are common enough during the early phase of carnivore that they should be expected rather than dramatized. You learned that rendered liquid fat can be harder for some people to tolerate than fat attached to the meat itself, and that a lower-residue diet naturally produces less stool without automatically meaning constipation. Instead of reacting to every digestive change as a problem, this chapter reframed digestion as a system adapting to new inputs, one that often improves with better meal structure, adequate hydration, proper sodium intake, and time.

From there, we addressed bloodwork and metabolic interpretation. Rather than treating a single lab value as a final verdict, you were shown how to read patterns with greater intelligence. We examined the Lean Mass Hyper-Responder phenotype, the debate around LDL elevation in carbohydrate-restricted states, and the importance of markers such as triglycerides, HDL, and the triglyceride-to-HDL ratio. At the same time, the chapter made clear that debate doesn't equal safety, and that rising LDL should be interpreted with caution, context, and, when appropriate, deeper evaluation. We also clarified the dawn phenomenon, showing that a mildly elevated fasting glucose in the morning may reflect normal hormonal fuel mobilization rather than dysfunction, especially when the broader pattern remains stable.

The chapter then turned to hormones, performance, and real life. For women, we emphasized that reproductive health is closely tied to getting enough food, recovering well, and managing stress. Under-eating, excessive fasting, and training too hard can create hormonal problems even within an otherwise well-designed diet. We also addressed the adaptive dip in exercise performance, explaining that many people experience a temporary loss of explosiveness, speed, or gym sharpness during the first few weeks as the body adjusts to a different fuel mix. We also acknowledged that sleep disruption can happen during the early transition and shouldn't automatically be treated as failure. The full explanation is reserved for Chapter 5, where sleep receives the dedicated attention, it deserves.

Finally, we dealt with social pressure and dining out. The point was simple, the greatest threat to consistency is often not biological. It's social. With a clear script, a practical ordering strategy, and a willingness to let other people be uncomfortable, carnivore becomes much easier to sustain outside the home.

Chapter 5: The Carnivore Lifestyle: Movement & Environment

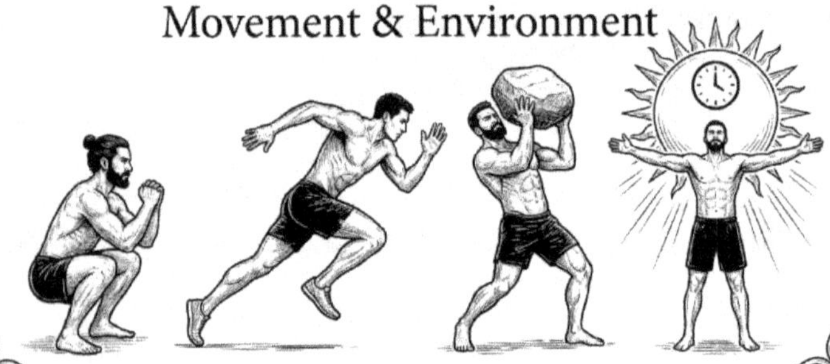

CHAPTER 5

THE CARNIVORE LIFESTYLE, MOVEMENT & ENVIRONMENT

Chapter 5 takes the carnivore framework beyond food and into the world your body lives in every day. Diet matters. Food can help reduce irritation, stabilize energy, and give the body the raw materials it needs to repair. But food alone can't fully rebuild a person who's living in an artificial environment. If the body is fed well but spends most of the day sitting in chairs, under artificial lights, away from sunlight, and disconnected from real movement, it can still remain weak, stiff, anxious, under-muscled, and metabolically incomplete.

That's because the human body doesn't respond only to nutrients. It also responds to signals. It adapts to posture, force, impact, speed, light, rhythm, and rest. Our ancestors didn't just eat animal foods. They also lived in ways that constantly told the body what it needed to become. They squatted, carried, walked, sprinted, climbed, lifted, rested, and rose with the sun. Those repeated signals helped build strong hips, durable bones, stable energy, and better alignment with the natural day-night cycle. When those signals disappear, the body starts to downshift.

This chapter is about restoring those missing signals. You'll learn why the deep squat matters as a basic human position, why sprinting and strength training send powerful muscle-building messages, why impact helps build stronger bones, why sunlight may be one of the most overlooked health inputs in modern life, and why sleep is the recovery signal that allows the rest of the system to work. The goal isn't to create an extreme training plan. The goal is to reconnect the body to the movement, light, and recovery patterns it was built to expect. If food is the fuel, this chapter is about the signals that tell the engine how to perform.

THE PRIMAL SQUAT: RESTORING THE DEFAULT SETTING

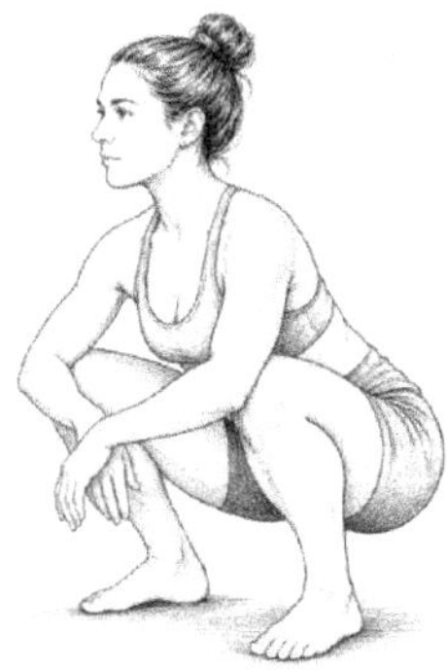

Modern life has trained the squat out of daily life. Most people wake up in a bed, sit down to get dressed, sit in a vehicle to drive, sit at a desk to work, and then sit again to eat, relax, and unwind. This constant time in chairs isn't a harmless convenience. It trains the body in the wrong direction. Over time, the body adapts to the positions it spends the most time in. The hips lose range of motion, the ankles get stiff, the glutes stop firing the way they should, and the lower back starts taking stress that should be shared by the hips, legs, and feet. What many people call aging is often just years of adapting to poor movement and bad positions.

The deep squat is different. It isn't just a gym exercise; it's a basic human resting position. It's one of the most natural positions the body can use when the joints still move the way they're supposed to. Babies drop into deep squats without being taught. Children do it naturally until chairs, modern shoes, and inactivity slowly train it out of them. In many traditional cultures, people still squat to rest, work, cook, and use the bathroom. The body recognizes this position as normal when it hasn't been trained away from it.

From a movement standpoint, the squat is a full-body maintenance position. It helps restore ankle mobility, hip mobility, and better knee control. It also reconnects the foot to the ground, which matters more than most people realize. When ankle mobility is lost, the body doesn't simply ignore the problem. It compensates. The knees may collapse inward, the heels may rise, the pelvis may tuck under, or the lower back may round too much. In plain language, when one joint stops doing its job, another area must pay the price. This is why stiff ankles, and tight hips can often show up as knee pain, back pain, or poor walking mechanics. The squat exposes these weaknesses quickly, and when practiced consistently, it can help improve them.

The squat also has an important nervous system benefit. It teaches the body how to relax while under tension. That may sound small, but it matters. Many people live with constant muscular guarding, tight hips, tight lower backs, clenched posture, and shallow breathing. Sitting all day can make that worse. A deep squat, when held calmly and breathed through, can help the body let go of some of that tension. It encourages the hips, pelvic floor, lower back, and ribcage to work together more naturally. Done properly, it isn't just a mobility drill. It's a reset for posture, breathing, and movement quality.

There may also be a practical digestive benefit. The human body often eliminates more efficiently in a squatting position than in a standard seated toilet position. Squatting changes the angle of the pelvis and rectum, which can make bowel movements easier and reduce the need to strain. That matters even more in a low-residue carnivore framework, where stool volume is naturally lower and people sometimes mistake going less often for a problem. A daily squat practice can help preserve the mechanics of elimination and reduce the stiff, stagnant feeling that often comes from years of chair-based living.

The key is to treat the squat as daily restoration, not as a test of toughness. You don't need to force a perfect rock-bottom squat on day one. In fact, forcing it too aggressively is one of the fastest ways to irritate a stiff body. Start where you are. Use a doorframe, countertop, or suspension strap for support. If your heels rise, place a small wedge, folded towel, or book under them. Let your body borrow the position before it earns it. Spend short periods at the bottom and focus on slow breathing while your hips, ankles, and feet adjust. Over time, the joints begin to open, the tissues become less defensive, and the squat starts to feel less like an exercise and more like a natural resting position.

A good starting goal is to build up to 5 minutes of squatting per day, then gradually work toward 10 to 15 minutes total. This doesn't need to happen all at once. You can squat for 30 seconds while waiting for food to heat, a minute while brushing your teeth, or several minutes during movement breaks throughout the day. The point is frequency. The body changes through repeated exposure, not heroic effort. Small, consistent doses retrain the system far better than occasional punishment sessions.

If you want more benefit, pair the squat with a few simple principles. Keep your feet planted as fully as you can. Let your knees move forward naturally instead of forcing them back. Keep your chest relaxed instead of trying to hold a stiff, perfect posture. Breathe into your belly instead of holding tension in your neck and shoulders. Think of the squat less like a stretch and more like feedback from your body. It shows you what's tight, what's weak, what's unstable, and where your body has been compensating.

In the larger carnivore framework, the primal squat represents something deeper than mobility. It's a return to a basic human posture that modern life has almost erased. It reminds the body that it was meant to move through full ranges of motion, rest close to the ground, and maintain joint function without constant artificial support. A person who can squat deeply, breathe calmly, and stand back up without strain is showing something more valuable than flexibility. He's showing retained function.

The primal squat isn't about looking athletic. It's about reclaiming a fundamental human position that helps preserve mobility, supports easier elimination, restores joint function, and reminds the body what it was built to do.

SPRINTING: THE HUNTER'S SIGNAL

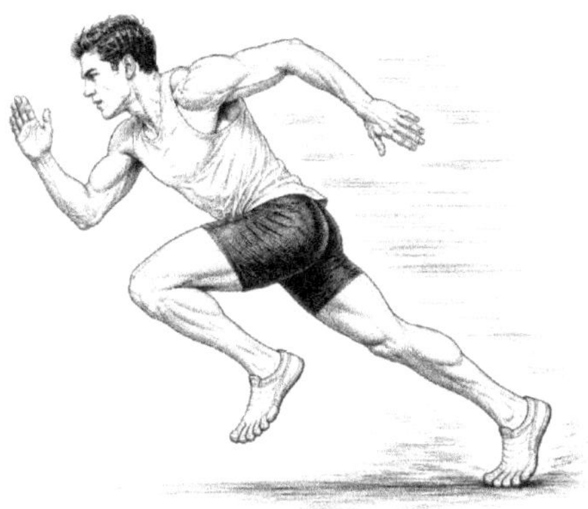

Humans aren't built to make endless, repetitive cardio the foundation of physical training. We're built for contrast, lots of low-intensity movement with short bursts of hard effort. That's the rhythm of the hunt. Walk. Track. Stalk. Then explode. Sprinting isn't just conditioning. It's a powerful biological signal. It tells the body that speed, power, coordination, and force still matter. In a world that trains most people to become soft, slow, and tired, sprinting sends the opposite message.

This is why sprinting gives you such a strong return for the time invested. Too much steady-state cardio can leave some people feeling depleted, especially when food, recovery, and sleep aren't handled well. Sprinting sends a different message. It tells the body to preserve strength, speed, and explosive ability. It puts a lot of demand on the muscles, tendons, lungs, heart, and nervous system in a very short amount of time. Instead of teaching the body to coast at a slow pace, sprinting teaches it to stay powerful, athletic, and ready.

From a hormone and performance standpoint, sprinting is one of the clearest ways to remind the body that it still has to perform. Short, hard efforts can support muscle-building signals, improve insulin sensitivity, and challenge the mitochondria, which are the energy-producing parts of the cells. Put simply, sprinting tells the body to keep its high-performance machinery. It's the difference between training only to last longer and training to produce force. One helps the body cover distance. The other helps the body accelerate, recover, and respond under pressure.

Sprinting also trains something modern life slowly weakens, nervous system sharpness. Most people live in a very narrow physical range. They sit, shuffle, stroll, and rarely ask the body to move with real urgency. Over time, the body adapts downward. Muscles stop firing as well. Tendons lose spring. Stride length gets shorter. Coordination becomes duller. Sprinting pushes back against that decline. It demands full-body coordination. The feet must strike well, the hips must drive, the arms must pump, the trunk must stay stable, and the brain must organize the whole movement in real time. Few movements restore athletic function this quickly.

There's also a mental effect that shouldn't be ignored. Sprinting requires commitment. You can't casually sprint. You either go or you don't. That alone makes it valuable. It trains intent. It teaches the body and mind to handle intensity. In that sense, sprinting is more than exercise, it's practice for decisive effort. It restores a quality that modern comfort slowly removes.

The plan doesn't need to be complicated. Two to three sessions per week is enough for most people, especially in the beginning. Perform 4 to 8 sprints of 10 to 20 seconds at near-maximal effort, with full recovery between efforts. Each sprint should be sharp, fast, and controlled. If your speed drops hard and your form falls apart, the session is over. Sprinting works best when the effort stays explosive, not when it turns into ugly survival shuffling.

Recovery is part of the training. Take enough rest between sprints so you can produce real effort in the next round. For some people, that may mean 60 to 90 seconds. For others, especially beginners, it may mean two or three minutes. Don't turn sprinting into punishment. The goal isn't to feel destroyed. The goal is to send a clear athletic signal to the body, be fast, be powerful, be resilient.

Safety matters here because sprinting is brutally honest. It exposes weakness quickly. If you haven't sprinted in years, don't start on a flat track trying to relive your high school glory days. Start with gentle hill sprints. A hill naturally shortens the stride, reduces impact, and may lower the risk of hamstring strain while still giving you the muscular and metabolic demand that makes sprinting useful. It also encourages better mechanics by making you drive the knees and push through the ground. In many cases, hill sprints are the safest reentry point for a deconditioned modern body.

Warm up properly before every session. Walk first. Loosen the ankles, hips, calves, and hamstrings. Perform a few controlled accelerations before attempting anything near maximal effort. Sprinting cold is reckless. The tissues need warning before they're asked to produce force at high speed. A few extra minutes of preparation can prevent weeks of setback. Save longer static stretching for after sprint training, not before.

It's also worth understanding what sprinting isn't. It isn't marathon training. It isn't a punishment for eating. It isn't a calorie-burning gimmick. It's a signal, a message to the body that explosiveness still matters. Within a carnivore framework, where you're already supplying high-quality protein and fat, sprinting provides a functional demand. It tells the body what to do with those nutrients: preserve muscle, improve power, maintain speed, and stay capable.

In the end, sprinting is one of the most efficient ways to reclaim your physical edge. It's brief, intense, and deeply human. It doesn't ask you to spend hours grinding yourself into the ground. It asks for a few moments of honest effort, delivered with intent. That's why it works. It speaks a language the body has always understood.

Sprinting is the hunter's signal, a brief and uncompromising reminder that the human body was built not merely to endure, but to explode.

HIIT: Bridging the Metabolic Gap

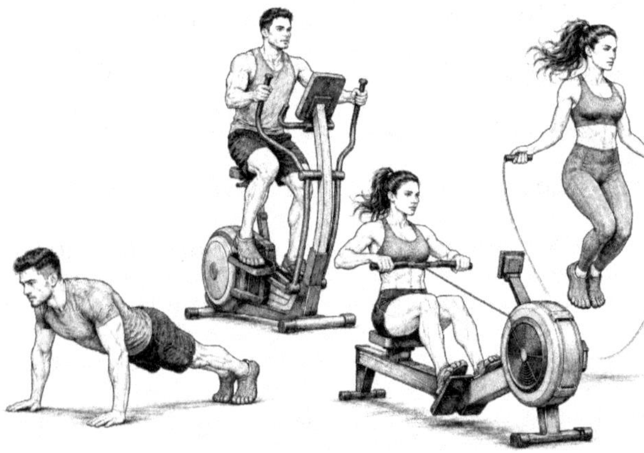

High-Intensity Interval Training, or HIIT, is one of the most efficient ways to condition the body for real life while still respecting the older pattern of human performance. It follows the rhythm of hard effort followed by recovery, push, recover, then push again. Sprinting is one form of interval training, but it deserves its own section because of how important and powerful it is. HIIT is broader. In practical terms, it trains your ability to surge, recover, and surge again. That matters because life rarely asks for perfectly paced effort. It asks you to handle repeated effort under imperfect conditions, climbing stairs quickly, chasing a child, carrying something heavy, responding under stress, or pushing hard when you're already somewhat tired.

This is where HIIT becomes valuable. It trains the body to handle intensity and recover from it instead of simply grinding through long, repetitive cardio. During a hard interval, the body has to produce energy quickly. Between intervals, the body works to recover, clear byproducts, restore breathing, and prepare for the next round. That back-and-forth is what makes HIIT effective. It doesn't train only one system. It forces several systems to work together under pressure, which is much closer to real human demand.

One of the key benefits of HIIT is that it can improve your ability to handle hard effort before you burn out. Lactate is often misunderstood in fitness culture. It isn't just a waste product to fear. It's part of how the body manages fuel during intense work. The real question isn't whether lactate shows up. It's how well your body can tolerate it, move it, and reuse it. HIIT can help improve that ability. It teaches the body how to work at higher intensities without falling apart right away. Over time, the same effort can feel less chaotic, recovery can become faster, and the body can become more adaptable.

Then there's EPOC, which stands for Excess Post-Exercise Oxygen Consumption. In plain language, HIIT makes the body keep working after the workout is over. Heart rate can stay elevated for a while, breathing may remain higher, and the body keeps working to return to normal. That means the training effect doesn't stop the second the session ends. HIIT can create a lingering demand as the body repairs, restores, and adapts.

But the value of HIIT isn't just about burning calories. That's a shallow way to look at it. HIIT teaches the heart to speed up and recover. It teaches the lungs to handle urgency. It teaches the muscles to work hard without immediate panic. It teaches the nervous system that discomfort is survivable and that effort can be repeated even when the body would rather coast. This kind of conditioning carries over beyond appearance. It improves work capacity, mental toughness, and the ability to perform in real life instead of only looking fit under controlled conditions.

Within a carnivore framework, HIIT becomes especially interesting. A fat-adapted person may experience energy differently than someone constantly riding the highs and lows of a carbohydrate-heavy diet. Without frequent blood sugar swings, the shift between hard effort and recovery may feel steadier and less erratic for some people. Many people report that they don't crash as hard between efforts and that recovery feels cleaner, steadier, and less dependent on immediate sugar. That doesn't mean HIIT becomes easy. It means the energy swings some people associate with hard interval training may be reduced when the body isn't depending on constant glucose hits.

This is what I'd call the carnivore advantage, steadier output, steadier recovery, and less drama between intervals. The body still uses glycogen for high-intensity work, but it may become better at managing energy overall. It can produce force when needed and then settle back into recovery without the same roller coaster effect that many people experience on a high-carbohydrate, low-satiety diet. In that sense, HIIT and carnivore can complement each other well. HIIT challenges metabolic flexibility, while carnivore may help stabilize the fuel system that supports it.

The practical application of HIIT doesn't need to be complicated. It can be done with sprint intervals, assault bikes, rowing machines, kettlebell swings, hill runs, or bodyweight circuits if the effort is truly intense. The structure is simple, short bursts of hard effort followed by partial recovery. For example, you might do 15 to 30 seconds of near-maximal work followed by 45 to 90 seconds of easier movement or rest. Repeat this for 6 to 10 rounds, depending on your conditioning. The key is honesty. If the work interval is too easy, it isn't HIIT. If the session drags on forever, it has turned into something else.

That said, HIIT is a powerful tool, not a daily requirement. Too much of it can become counterproductive. Two to three sessions per week is enough for most people. More than that can turn intensity into chronic stress, especially if sleep, recovery, and overall life stress aren't being managed well. A carnivore lifestyle should make you more robust, not more depleted.

Technique and exercise selection matter here as well. Choose movements you can perform hard without falling apart. A bike sprint is safer for many people than all-out burpees with collapsing form. A hill sprint may be smarter than repeated flat-ground sprints for someone with poor mechanics. The training should be hard, but not reckless. There's no prize for injury. The point is adaptation and fitness.

In the broader context of this chapter, HIIT serves as a bridge. It sits between pure endurance and pure strength, between low-intensity movement and all-out explosive effort. It fills the metabolic gap by training the body to operate in the middle ground where life often happens, not resting, not all-out, but repeatedly called upon to perform. It helps transform the body from something that only handles one speed into something that can shift gears on command.

LIFTING HEAVY THINGS

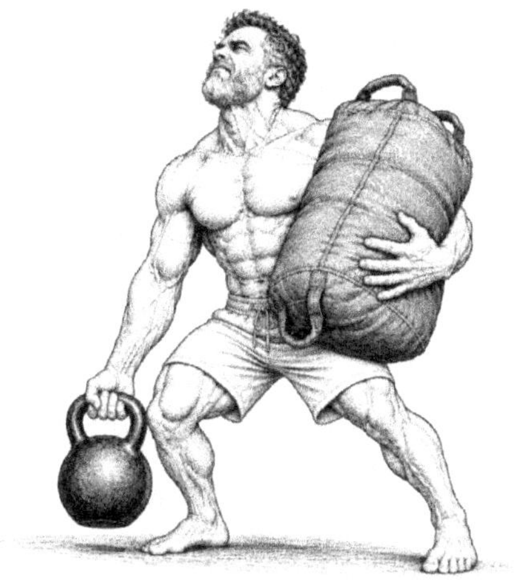

On a carnivore approach, you're giving your body highly usable protein, essential fats, cholesterol, creatine, carnitine, iron, zinc, and fat-soluble nutrients that support repair and adaptation. But nutrients alone don't decide what the body builds. The body responds to demand. Strength training provides that demand. It gives your nutrition a job. Without the signal of resistance, your body has less reason to use those raw materials to build muscle, connective tissue, and strong bones.

This is why lifting matters so much. It isn't just about appearance, vanity, or chasing numbers in the gym. It's about telling the body what kind of organism it still needs to be. A body that's never challenged will slowly downshift. It'll lose strength, lose muscle, reduce work capacity, and become structurally weaker over time. That decline is often called normal aging. In many cases, it isn't just age causing the decline. It's the lack of a meaningful strength signal.

Muscle should be viewed as one of the body's most important assets for aging well. It helps the body handle glucose, supports insulin sensitivity, protects metabolic health, improves balance and coordination, and gives you physical reserve as you get older. A stronger person is harder to break. He's more resilient to injury, more stable under fatigue, and better prepared to handle stress, illness, and the demands of life.

And muscle never works alone. When you lift heavy loads, you aren't only training muscle. You're also training tendons, ligaments, fascia, and bone. Bone responds to the force placed on it. If you give the body repeated, appropriate resistance, it responds by building a stronger frame. If you remove that demand, the body starts to conserve resources. Bones become less robust, connective tissue weakens, and posture can deteriorate. Strength training is structural. It reinforces the entire body.

The most productive way to train isn't through endless machine circuits or random exercises. The body responds best to foundational movement patterns compound, multi-joint lifts that require coordination, stability, and multiple muscle groups working together. These movements look more like real-life strength. The deadlift teaches you to hinge, brace, and lift from the hips. The squat builds leg strength, pelvic control, and structural resilience. The overhead press trains shoulder strength, trunk stability, and force transfer through the whole body. The loaded carry may be the most honest movement of all, pick up something heavy and move with it. Carries train grip, posture, breathing, core stability, and practical strength that matters outside the gym.

There's a reason these movements have lasted. They work. They use a lot of muscle, create a strong demand on the body, and send a clear signal for adaptation. They also expose weakness quickly. A person can hide behind easy isolation exercises for years and still remain fragile. He can't hide under a heavy barbell or while carrying a heavy load across the room. Compound lifts reveal what's strong, what's unstable, and what still needs work.

Within a carnivore framework, lifting becomes even more powerful. If sprinting is the signal for explosiveness, lifting is the signal for structure. It tells the body to preserve and build the machinery needed to produce force. The amino acids from meat aren't just food, they become the building blocks for muscle tissue. The fat and cholesterol you eat aren't just energy, they help support hormone production, recovery, and cellular repair. Lifting gives those nutrients a clear job.

This is why training volume has to be managed intelligently. More isn't always better. Daily hard sessions that leave you constantly fatigued can interfere with recovery, especially if they become nothing more than accumulated wear and tear. Three to four focused strength sessions per week, around 45 minutes each, is usually more productive than six or seven mediocre sessions that keep the body in a constant state of low-grade exhaustion. Quality matters more than quantity. Recovery is where the adaptation happens, and anyone training hard should respect that.

A good strength session should feel focused, not chaotic. Pick a few key movements, do them well, and leave. There's no prize for turning the gym into a three-hour endurance event. The goal is to send a clear message to the body, preserve muscle, strengthen the frame, improve force production, and then recover. Brief, heavy, intentional work usually beats scattered effort.

Progressive overload is the main principle. The body keeps adapting only when the challenge continues to rise in some way. That doesn't always mean adding more weight every session. It can mean improving form, adding a repetition, controlling the movement better, increasing range of motion, or carrying the same weight with better posture and control. The body doesn't care about gym culture. It cares whether the challenge is strong enough to require adaptation.

Technique matters because heavy lifting is only helpful when the force is organized well. A deadlift with a loose brace and poor hip hinge isn't productive strength training. It's a setup for compensation and injury. The same applies to the squat, the press, and the carry. Learn the movement first. Own the pattern. Then add load. Strength built on poor mechanics is unstable strength, and unstable strength eventually breaks down under pressure.

There's also a psychological benefit to lifting that shouldn't be underestimated. Heavy resistance training teaches composure under load. It demands attention, breathing, discipline, and controlled aggression. In that sense, it isn't only building the body. It's also training the nervous system and the mindset required to handle stress.

For beginners, simplicity is the advantage. You don't need a complicated split routine or an elaborate spreadsheet to benefit. Start with the basic movements. Learn to squat. Learn to press. Learn to pull. Learn to carry. Train them consistently, recover properly, and let time do its work. For older adults or people returning after years of inactivity, even bodyweight squats, kettlebell deadlifts, dumbbell carries, and simple presses can provide a major benefit. The principle is the same regardless of the tool, the body must feel resistance if it's going to remain strong.

In the long term, lifting heavy things is one of the clearest ways to resist physical decline. It helps preserve muscle mass, reinforce bone, support metabolic health, sharpen the nervous system, and give your carnivore nutrition a clear purpose. You aren't just eating to survive. You're eating to build a body that can produce force, absorb stress, and remain useful.

SKELETAL IMPACT: BUILDING STRONGER BONES

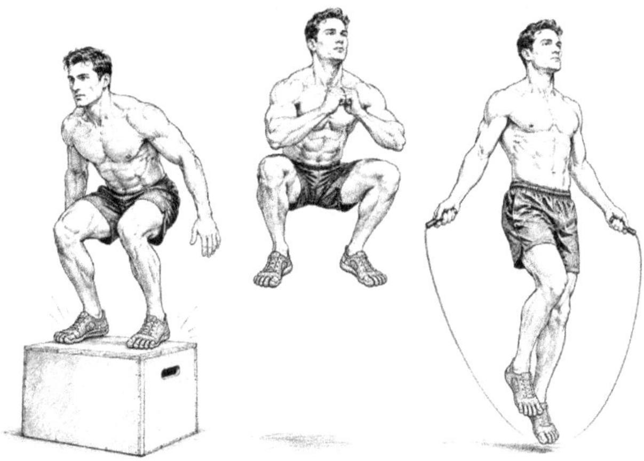

Modern life has quietly removed one of the most important signals the body needs, impact. We walk on carpet, polished floors, rubber gym surfaces, and concrete softened by thick shoes. We sit more, jump less, and rarely ask the skeleton to absorb real force. The result is predictable. Bones, joints, tendons, and feet receive less of the mechanical stress they were built to handle. Over time, the body adapts to that lack of stress. The frame becomes weaker, less responsive, and more fragile. What many people call normal aging is often the long-term result of an underused skeleton.

Bone isn't dead scaffolding. It's living tissue that constantly changes based on the forces placed on it. If the skeleton is exposed to the right amount of force, it responds by becoming stronger and more resilient. If that force disappears, the body has less reason to keep the structure strong. In that sense, impact isn't abuse when it's applied properly. It's information. It's a signal that tells the body the frame still needs to handle landing, jumping, running, sudden movement, and changes in direction.

Impact matters because it gives the body a kind of signal that ordinary walking and machine-based exercise often don't provide. When your foot hits the ground with enough force, that force travels through the feet, ankles, lower legs, thighs, hips, and spine. That signal helps tell the skeleton to stay strong. Without it, the body gets a weaker message. You may still move, but the frame may not get enough reason to toughen itself. Controlled impact restores that message.

This doesn't mean you should recklessly start jumping off boxes or sprinting barefoot on asphalt. That isn't training. That's impatience. The body must be prepared in layers. Progression matters. Start with low-level impact that brings force back without overwhelming the tissues. Heel drops are a simple starting point. So are jumping jacks, light hops in place, or controlled step-downs from a low surface. These drills wake up the feet, calves, Achilles tendons, and lower legs while teaching the body to handle force again. Once that becomes easy and pain-free, you can move to skipping, low pogo jumps, and small step-offs. Only after months of consistent adaptation should higher-impact work like vertical jumps, bounding, or barefoot running be considered.

Modern people often have strong ambition sitting on top of weak tissues. That's a dangerous combination. Your muscles may feel ready long before your tendons, fascia, feet, and bones are prepared. Impact training punishes impatience. Done too aggressively, it can lead to shin splints, Achilles irritation, plantar fascia pain, or joint flare-ups. Done gradually, it can do the opposite. It can strengthen the lower body and rebuild your ability to meet the ground with confidence instead of collapse.

This is where the feet become extremely important. The foot isn't just a block at the end of the leg. It's a dynamic, sensory-rich structure built to absorb force, stabilize the body, and send information to the brain. Each foot contains many joints, muscles, tendons, and sensors that help the body understand the ground. When the foot is allowed to work properly, it acts as both a shock absorber and a communication system. When it's trapped for years in stiff, heavily cushioned shoes, much of that function can become weaker. The foot may become less responsive, less strong, and less able to handle uneven ground or dynamic movement.

Barefoot Mechanics and Controlled Impact

Barefoot mechanics can help restore some of the foot function that modern life has weakened. When done safely and gradually, barefoot training can help rebuild proprioception. Proprioception is the body's ability to sense where it is in space. Your feet are supposed to send constant information to your brain about the ground, your balance, and how your body is moving.

Modern cushioned shoes can interfere with that feedback. When thick padding blocks the foot from feeling the ground, the body may move with less precision. People may land harder, move less efficiently, and lose some of the quick adjustments the feet are supposed to make. In many cases, the more padding you put between yourself and the ground, the less clearly your body can read the surface beneath you.

But the goal isn't to throw away your shoes overnight and pretend your feet are ready for full barefoot living. That isn't toughness. That's stupidity. The goal is reconditioning. Start indoors by spending more time barefoot around the house. Let the toes spread. Let the arches begin to work again. Let the foot relearn how to grip, stabilize, and respond without constant artificial support. As tolerance improves, move to short outdoor walks in minimalist or barefoot-style shoes that allow more natural movement while still protecting your feet from sharp surfaces. Build slowly. Weak feet don't become strong through one dramatic effort. They become strong through frequent, manageable exposure.

As the feet improve, everything above them can improve too. Stronger feet may help with balance, ankle stability, walking mechanics, and force transfer through the knees and hips. The arch can begin working more like a spring again. The calves can regain some of their natural elasticity. Posture may improve because the body is receiving clearer information from the ground. This is why foot strength isn't a small side issue. It's foundational. A weak, numb, unstable foot can affect the entire chain above it.

Skeletal impact training also has a psychological effect. People who are disconnected from the ground often move with caution, stiffness, and hesitation. Their bodies have lost trust in their own structure. Reintroducing controlled impact, along with foot strengthening and better ground contact, can help restore that trust. You begin to feel less brittle, less hesitant, and more capable of landing, absorbing force, and moving with spring instead of collapse. That quality matters, especially as the years go on. Resilience isn't only about muscle. It's also about how well the frame itself can handle life.

Within the carnivore framework, this matters because diet provides the raw materials, but impact provides the instruction. Animal foods give the body protein, minerals, fat-soluble vitamins, and the nutritional building blocks for repair. Controlled impact tells the skeleton what to do with those resources. It tells the body that bones need to stay strong, connective tissue needs to stay durable, and the lower body needs to remain capable of handling force. Without that signal, even strong nutrition can't fully express itself through the body's structure.

In practical terms, think of skeletal impact as one of the missing signals of modern life. Not reckless impact. Not chronic pounding. Controlled, progressive, intelligent impact. Enough to wake the frame up. Enough to tell the body it still needs to be strong.

Bones become stronger not by being protected from every impact, but by being exposed to the right amount of impact in the right way.

SOLAR NUTRITION

Food is a biological input, but light is one of the body's master signals. You can eat the cleanest diet in the world and still feel tired, anxious, hormonally off, mentally flat, or poorly recovered if your daily light rhythm is broken. The human body doesn't run only on calories and nutrients. It also runs on timing. It needs to know when it's day, when it's night, when to be alert, when to produce hormones, when to digest, and when to repair. Light, especially natural outdoor light, is the main signal that helps organize that timing.

Your circadian rhythm isn't some fringe wellness idea. It's one of the body's main operating systems. It affects cortisol release, melatonin production, insulin sensitivity, body temperature, immune activity, hunger signals, mood, and sleep quality. When that rhythm is lined up properly, many systems work better with less effort. When it's disrupted, the body becomes less organized. You may still function, but it often comes with more cravings, worse sleep, poorer recovery, lower energy, and less resilience.

This is why morning sunlight matters so much. Getting outdoor light shortly after waking, ideally within the first thirty minutes, helps set the body's internal clock. This isn't about staring at the sun. It's about getting outside and letting natural light reach your eyes without a window filtering it. Morning light tells the brain that the day has begun. That signal helps regulate the morning cortisol rhythm, improves alertness, and starts the countdown for melatonin release later that night. In plain language, the quality of your sleep tonight can begin with the light you see this morning.

That one habit can have a major effect. A person who gets morning sunlight consistently may notice steadier energy, better mood, clearer appetite signals, and an easier time falling asleep at night. This happens because the body is no longer guessing what time it is. It has been given a clear signal. Modern indoor living weakens that signal. Most people wake up under dim artificial light, spend the day inside under weak indoor lighting, and then blast their eyes with screens and bright overhead lights at night. To the nervous system, that's confusion.

Sunlight also affects the skin in ways that go beyond vitamin D. Sunlight on the skin helps the body make vitamin D and may influence other processes related to immune function, inflammation control, and biological rhythm. The skin isn't just a covering. It's a light-responsive organ. Sun exposure isn't only about avoiding deficiency. It's about giving the body an environmental signal it was built to receive regularly.

This matters because modern people often try to supplement their way out of an environmental problem. A vitamin D pill may help in some situations, but it isn't the same as receiving the full signal from actual sunlight. Natural light provides timing, brightness, color variation, and environmental context that a capsule can't copy. That doesn't mean standing outside for ten minutes fixes everything. It means the body expects sunlight as part of normal life, and when that input is missing for too long, function can suffer.

Artificial light at night is the other side of the problem. If morning sunlight tells the body to wake up, bright artificial light after sunset tells the body to stay awake when it should be winding down. Phones, tablets, televisions, and bright overhead lights can stretch the biological day far beyond what the brain expects. This can suppress melatonin, delay sleep, reduce sleep quality, and weaken recovery. The result isn't just a rough night. It can also mean more hunger the next day, worse blood sugar control, irritability, reduced training capacity, and a body that feels overstimulated.

This is why dimming your environment after sunset isn't a gimmick. It's recovery. Lower the lights. Reduce screen exposure. Use lamps instead of overhead lighting when possible. Avoid blasting your eyes with bright white or blue-heavy light late at night. You don't need to become obsessive, but you do need to respect the biology. A darker environment at night is just as important as bright light in the morning.

Think of sunlight and darkness as information for the nervous system. Morning light tells the body to wake up, become alert, move, and prepare hormonally for the day. Evening darkness tells the body to slow down, repair, recover, and shift toward a calmer state. When those signals are clear, sleep often improves. When sleep improves, everything else tends to get easier, hunger becomes more stable, cravings decrease, mood steadies, training recovery improves, and the body is better able to regulate stress. In that sense, sleep isn't just rest. It's repair. It's where much of the rebuilding happens.

Within a carnivore framework, this becomes especially important. A nutrient-dense, low-noise diet may reduce many of the food-related burdens that interfere with health. But if the nervous system remains trapped in circadian confusion from too little daylight, too much indoor living, and too much bright light at night, recovery remains incomplete. You may clean up the food and still feel like something is missing. Often, what's missing isn't another supplement or a stricter diet. It's better alignment with the environment your body expects.

The practical application is simple, even if the effects can be powerful. Get outside early. Seek natural light in the morning. Let your eyes receive outdoor light without staring at the sun. Expose your skin to daylight regularly when appropriate. Move your body outdoors when possible. As evening approaches, reduce artificial light and create a darker, quieter environment. Protect sleep with the same seriousness you protect your diet. The body can't fully recover in a light environment that keeps sending mixed signals.

In the end, solar nutrition is about respecting an ancient truth, the human body evolved under the sun, not under LED panels and glowing screens. Light isn't just background. It's one of the major signals that helps govern life itself.

SLEEP: THE RECOVERY SIGNAL

Every protocol in this book depends on sleep to deliver its results. The sprints you ran, the steaks you ate, the fasting window you maintained, and the heavy lifts you performed with discipline and intent don't fully pay off while you're awake. They pay off while you sleep. Sleep isn't a passive gap between productive hours. It's one of the most important recovery periods in the twenty-four-hour cycle. It's when growth hormone rises, tissue repair increases, the nervous system resets, and the body processes the demands of the day. If sleep is too short, too broken, or too shallow for too long, you aren't just tired. You're weakening every other part of this framework.

This is what makes sleep so important in the context of carnivore. Most people understand that sleep matters in a general way. Far fewer understand that sleep is where many of the benefits from food, training, sunlight, and recovery actually get organized. If you're eating well, moving intelligently, and getting enough sunlight, but still sleeping poorly, you're leaving results on the table every night. The body doesn't care how clean your diet is if it's being denied the time it needs to repair, regulate, and rebuild.

Sleep as a Hormonal Event

The most important thing to understand about sleep is that it isn't just rest. It's a hormonal event. The body doesn't simply pause during sleep. It shifts into a different operating mode, one that can't be fully replaced by supplements, caffeine, discipline, or willpower.

Growth hormone is released mostly during the deeper stages of sleep. That matters because growth hormone helps support tissue repair, fat metabolism, and muscle maintenance. If you're eating high-quality animal protein and training hard, sleep is part of how the body uses those inputs properly. Chronically poor sleep can weaken that recovery signal, which means the protein you ate and the training you did aren't being supported as well as they could be. You can't fully supplement your way around that. Sleep is part of the mechanism.

Cortisol also follows a daily rhythm that's closely tied to sleep. Under normal conditions, cortisol is lower during the early part of sleep and rises toward morning, helping the body prepare to wake up and function. When sleep is consistently too short or disrupted, that rhythm can become less stable. Cortisol may stay higher at times when it should be lower, which can affect blood sugar, insulin sensitivity, fat storage, and nervous system stress. In plain language, poor sleep can quietly work against many of the metabolic improvements you're trying to create.

Leptin and ghrelin are also affected by sleep. Leptin is connected to fullness and energy balance. Ghrelin is connected to hunger and appetite. Poor sleep can push those signals in the wrong direction, less fullness, more hunger, and stronger cravings, especially for high-reward foods. For someone trying to stabilize appetite and reduce food noise, poor sleep is one of the strongest forces working against that goal. You can eat well and still feel driven to keep eating if your sleep is consistently poor.

THE CARNIVORE-SPECIFIC SLEEP STORY

There's a sleep story specific to this way of eating that most people never hear, and it has two parts.

The first part is what can happen during the transition. In the first two to four weeks of carnivore, some people experience disrupted sleep. They may fall asleep easily but wake up in the middle of the night. They may have unusually vivid dreams. They may feel lighter, less rested, or oddly alert at strange hours. This doesn't automatically mean the diet is failing. It's often part of the same electrolyte shifts and metabolic adjustment discussed earlier. Changes in sodium, magnesium, insulin rhythm, and fuel use can all affect sleep temporarily. Adequate sodium, adequate magnesium, and enough total food often help. So does patience. For many people, this phase improves as adaptation progresses.

The second part is what can happen after adaptation, and this is where the carnivore framework may offer a real advantage for some people. Blood sugar stability during the night is one of the most overlooked parts of sleep quality. Some people wake at two or three in the morning not because of noise, but because their body is responding to a shift in blood sugar and stress hormones. On a carbohydrate-heavy diet with frequent insulin swings, nighttime glucose changes may be more noticeable. On a stable, fat-adapted diet, some people experience fewer of those disruptions. When the body becomes better at using fat and ketones for fuel, there may be fewer metabolic triggers waking the system during the night. Many people report that their sleep becomes deeper and more consistent once full adaptation arrives.

SLEEP APNEA AS A METABOLIC CONDITION

Sleep apnea deserves direct attention because it isn't always just a simple airway problem. In many people, it's closely tied to metabolic health. Sleep apnea is often linked with insulin resistance, excess body fat, visceral fat around the abdomen and organs, inflammation, and broader metabolic dysfunction. That's why sleep apnea may improve when metabolic health improves.

As body fat decreases, especially visceral fat, there may be less mechanical pressure around the airway. As inflammation improves, tissues may become less swollen or reactive. Better metabolic health may also support better breathing regulation during sleep. This doesn't mean carnivore cures sleep apnea. Severe sleep apnea, or sleep apnea caused by structural issues, still needs proper medical evaluation and treatment. But the connection between metabolic health and sleep apnea severity is real, and it's one more reason this framework reaches beyond food alone.

THE PRACTICAL FOUNDATION

Sleep quality is shaped by several practical habits that fit naturally with the carnivore lifestyle. Meal timing matters. Eating too close to bedtime can raise body temperature, increase digestive workload, and make it harder to fall asleep. The eating-window guidance discussed in Chapter 8 fits well here. Finishing your final meal two to three hours before bed gives the body time to handle the active part of digestion before the deeper recovery phase begins.

Magnesium glycinate deserves a practical place in this discussion. Many people eating a carnivore diet find it useful for supporting sleep quality and reducing nighttime muscle cramps, especially during the transition phase. A common starting range is 200 to 400 milligrams before bed. It isn't a magic fix, and it won't overcome a broken sleep environment, poor light habits, or chronic stress. But it can be a useful tool when magnesium intake or retention is low, and it may help support the deeper sleep quality needed for recovery.

Consistent sleep timing also matters. The body's internal clock responds to routine. Going to bed and waking up at roughly the same time each day, even on weekends, helps reinforce the rhythm that morning sunlight starts. Evening light management, covered in the Solar Nutrition section, is the other half of that rhythm. Morning light tells the body when the day begins. Evening darkness tells the body when to wind down. Together, they help create the conditions for deeper, more complete sleep.

Sleep Is Where the Work Pays Off

The larger principle is simple. You can't out-train poor sleep. You can't out-eat it. You can't fast your way past it or supplement around it. Sleep is the environment where every other input is processed. Without enough quality sleep, the return on everything else is reduced. A person eating a clean carnivore diet, training intelligently, managing stress, and getting sunlight, but sleeping five or six broken hours a night, isn't running a complete system. He's leaving the most important recovery window mostly unused.

Protect sleep with the same seriousness you protect your food. Give it structure. Give it darkness. Give it consistency. Give it enough total time. When the body finally gets what it needs from sleep, everything else in this framework starts to compound in a way that no single meal, supplement, or training session can match by itself.

A Note on Everything This Chapter Does Not Cover

Chapter 5 isn't a complete guide to exercise. It was never meant to be. The movements and practices described here, the squat, the sprint, interval work, heavy lifting, impact training, sunlight, and sleep, were chosen because the evidence and real-world experience behind them suggest they offer a strong return for the time and effort invested.

That means there's a lot this chapter didn't discuss. It didn't cover swimming, cycling, yoga, pickleball, recreational sports, group fitness classes, hiking, dancing, rowing, martial arts, or the many other physical activities people enjoy and benefit from. That omission isn't an accident, and it isn't a silent judgment. It's a choice about scope. This chapter gives you the highest-leverage tools. What you do with the rest of your physical life is up to you.

If you're sedentary right now, ignore most of what this chapter asks of you for the moment and start with one thing, walk. Walk outside if you can. Walk in the morning if your schedule allows. Walk after meals. Walk without your phone if you're willing. Walking isn't a consolation prize for people who aren't ready for "real exercise." It's one of the most underrated metabolic and mental health tools available. It can help support blood sugar control, reduce stress, reinforce circadian rhythm, and remind the body that it's still meant to move through the world under its own power. Many people who begin this way of eating from a sedentary place find that walking is the first domino. It's enough to start with. For many people, it's more than enough.

Beyond walking, do what you genuinely enjoy. Movement you'll actually do consistently beats the theoretically perfect plan you quit after three weeks. If you love hiking, hike. If lifting weights excites you, lift. If you play tennis, play tennis. If group classes keep you accountable, go to the class. Physical activity you look forward to isn't inferior to physical activity that looks better on paper. Enjoyment is part of sustainability, and sustainability is what produces results over years instead of weeks.

What this chapter argued, and what I believe based on my own experience and the best available evidence, is that certain inputs give the body unusually clear and powerful signals for a relatively small investment of time. Sprinting briefly and intelligently. Lifting heavy things with good form a few times per week. Relearning how to squat. Adding controlled impact. Moving barefoot. Getting morning light. Sleeping properly. These are the practices I return to because they consistently produce the clearest return. They aren't the only things that matter. They're the ones I'd choose first if time and energy were limited.

The goal of this chapter was never to make movement feel like another burden. The goal was to reconnect the body to demands it was built to meet, so that the food you're eating has somewhere purposeful to go. However, you choose to do that, whether through the practices described here or through something entirely your own, the body rewards consistency and genuine effort.

Move in the way that makes your life better. That's the standard that matters most in the long run.

SUMMARY OF CHAPTER 5

In this chapter, we moved beyond the plate and into the larger world that shapes whether a person merely survives or actually becomes strong. The carnivore diet strips away nutritional noise, reduces dietary friction, and supplies the raw materials for repair, but food alone isn't the full equation. The body is shaped by signals. It responds to movement, force, impact, light, rhythm, and rest. Remove those signals, and even a well-fed body can begin to soften, weaken, and drift. Modern life has made many people overfed, under-muscled, under-sunned, sleep-deprived, and physically disconnected from the demands that once built durable men and women. This chapter was about restoring those missing signals.

We began by reclaiming the Primal Squat, a forgotten resting posture that can help restore mobility, support easier elimination, and reintroduce the body to its natural mechanics. We then turned to sprinting, HIIT, and heavy lifting, forms of effort that clearly tell the body that speed, force, muscle, and recovery still matter. These practices help instruct the body to preserve strength, maintain power, build work capacity, and remain harder to break. We also addressed skeletal impact and barefoot mechanics, recognizing that bones, tendons, and feet don't become resilient through constant comfort and protection. They become stronger through intelligent exposure to load, contact, and force. A strong frame isn't inherited once and kept forever. It's earned and re-earned through stress the body is allowed to adapt to.

From there, we examined Solar Nutrition and the role of light in human health. Sunlight isn't just part of the scenery. It's one of the major signals that helps regulate hormones, energy, appetite, mood, and the body's internal clock. When morning light is missing and artificial light dominates the night, the body can lose its rhythm and pay for it with poor recovery, metabolic confusion, and a nervous system that can't fully wind down. Light is the instruction that tells the body what time it is and what it should be preparing to do.

Finally, we addressed sleep as the recovery signal that completes the entire framework. Every sprint, every heavy lift, and every well-built carnivore meal depends on sleep to deliver its full return. Sleep is where the body repairs tissue, supports hormone rhythms, restores nervous system balance, and processes the demands of the day. You learned that the transition phase can temporarily disrupt sleep and that this doesn't automatically mean the diet is failing. You also learned that full adaptation may improve sleep quality for some people as nighttime energy stability improves. Sleep apnea was addressed not as a simple airway issue alone, but as a condition often connected to metabolic health, insulin resistance, excess body fat, and visceral fat. In many people, improving metabolic health may help improve sleep apnea severity, though proper medical evaluation and treatment still matter.

The chapter closed with an honest acknowledgment of what it didn't cover. The practices described here were chosen for their return on investment, not because they're the only valid forms of movement. If you're sedentary, walking is a legitimate and underrated starting point, not a lesser option. If you love a form of movement this chapter never mentioned, do it. Enjoyment and consistency matter more than theoretical perfection. The squat, the sprint, the heavy lift, the impact work, the light, and the sleep were presented because they deliver strong signals for a relatively small investment of time. They are the inputs worth protecting first. They aren't the only inputs that count.

Chapter 6: The Ketovore Bridge & Transition Tools

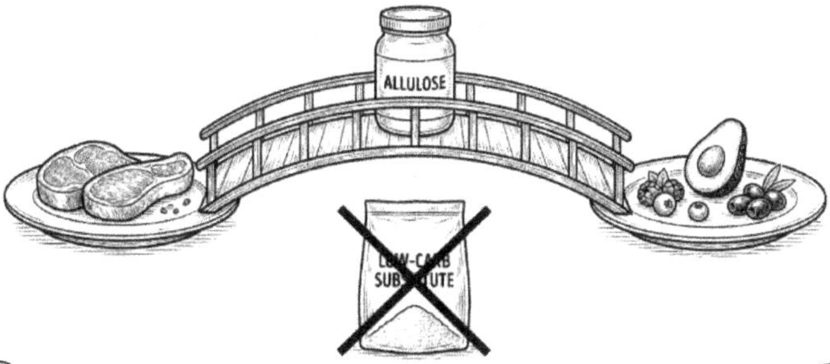

CHAPTER 6

THE KETOVORE BRIDGE & TRANSITION TOOLS

A strict carnivore framework aims for maximum clarity by removing as many dietary variables as possible. But not everyone transitions well by going from a lifetime of processed food, constant sweetness, and habitual carbohydrates straight into beef, salt, and water. For some people, that hard cut works. For others, it creates enough mental resistance, social pressure, or early instability that the entire plan collapses before the body ever has a chance to settle. That doesn't mean strict carnivore is wrong. It means transition strategy matters.

This chapter introduces the ketovore bridge as a controlled tool, not a compromise in principle. It exists for the person who needs a narrower, more strategic path between the Standard American Diet and a cleaner animal-based foundation. That may mean limited use of low-sugar plant foods, temporary use of a carefully chosen sweetener, or a fallback option that prevents a full relapse into processed junk. The point isn't to rebuild the old diet with cleaner branding. The point is to create just enough flexibility to stay consistent while still protecting metabolic stability.

The standard throughout this chapter is simple, anything added must earn its place. Added foods should reduce friction without reigniting cravings, raising the carbohydrate load too high, or bringing back the behavioral chaos of the old system. Used correctly, the ketovore bridge can help a person keep moving without losing the direction of travel. Used carelessly, it becomes a comfortable excuse to camp halfway. This chapter is about knowing the difference.

THE PLANT LIST: NAVIGATING LOW-TOXICITY WHOLE FOODS

If you choose to include plants in your protocol, they should enter as controlled variables, not as a return to dietary chaos. The purpose of strategic plant use isn't to rebuild the modern plate. It's to add limited flexibility, flavor, texture, or fermentation while preserving the metabolic stability you worked to create. That means the plants you choose should be low in sugar, modest in total carbohydrate, and easy to remove again if symptoms return. In this framework, plants aren't the foundation. They're optional extras.

The practical rule is carbohydrate control. Many ketogenic frameworks define very low-carbohydrate intake in the range of roughly 20 to 40 grams per day, and a cap around 30 grams of net carbohydrate can be a reasonable practical target for someone trying to preserve fat adaptation while experimenting with a small amount of plant food. It isn't a magic number, but it's a useful guardrail. Once intake starts drifting higher, especially through fruit, "healthy" snacks, or keto-branded treats, the metabolic simplicity of the protocol starts to erode.

That's why the plant list should be organized by function. Some foods behave more like fat sources than carbohydrate sources. Some can work as small garnish foods without creating major disruption. Others are only worth using if they're carefully prepared and clearly tolerated. The point isn't to romanticize plants. The point is to rank them according to how little trouble they're likely to cause.

- **Tier 1: Fat-Dominant Fruits**

Some botanical fruits act more like fat sources than sweet foods. These are often the easiest "bridge foods" because they provide texture, flavor, and fullness without adding much sugar. Avocado is the clearest example. It's rich in monounsaturated fat and potassium, and normal servings are usually fairly low in net carbohydrates. Olives work in a similar way, especially when they're simply brined instead of packed in seed-oil-heavy marinades or dressings. Unsweetened coconut meat can also fit here because it provides fat and some medium-chain triglycerides, though portions still matter. Carb counts can vary by product and preparation, so USDA Food Data Central is a useful place to check exact values when needed.

The practical value of this tier is that these foods can add variety without acting like dessert. They're usually easier to portion, easier to remove if symptoms return, and less likely to trigger the "just one more" pattern that sweeter foods often create. If someone wants a controlled starting point for adding plant foods, this is where I'd begin. Choose organic when possible, but don't let perfect sourcing become another excuse to delay action.

Food	**Portion**	**Net Carbs**	**Notes**
Avocado	½ medium	~2 g	High potassium; strong satiety

Olives	10 large	~1 g	Choose brined, not marinated
Coconut meat	½ cup (raw)	~3 g	Source of MCTs; avoid sweetened

- **Tier 2: Low-Sugar Berries**

Berries sit in the middle. They're still fruit, and they still contain carbohydrates, but they're usually lower in sugar than many modern fruits. They work best as accents, not staples. A few berries once in a while is very different from a daily smoothie or a large bowl of fruit being treated as "clean eating." The issue isn't that berries exist. The issue is portion size and frequency.

Among common berries, blackberries and raspberries are usually the easiest fit in a low-carbohydrate plan because they tend to be lower in net carbohydrates than fruits like bananas, grapes, or mangoes. Strawberries can also fit in small amounts. Blueberries tend to contain more carbohydrates per serving and are easier to overeat, which is why they're often less useful during stricter transition phases.

Exact carbohydrate values depend on portion size, ripeness, product type, and the specific food entry used, so it's better to think in terms of "small garnish servings" instead of relying too heavily on one static chart.

Food	**Portion**	**Net Carbs**	**Notes**
Blackberries	½ cup	~3 g	Lowest sugar content
Raspberries	½ cup	~3.5 g	Tart; fiber-heavy
Strawberries	4 medium	~3 g	Buy organic if possible
Blueberries	½ cup	~11 g	Avoid during transition

- **Tier 3: Low-Toxicity Vegetables**

Vegetables are where precision matters most because the category is too broad to treat as one thing. Some vegetables are relatively low in sugar and may be tolerated in small amounts. Others bring more fiber, more fermentable carbohydrate, or more plant defense compounds than is useful in this framework. The stronger principle isn't "all vegetables are toxic." The stronger principle is that plants contain a wide range of compounds that can affect digestion, absorption, and tolerance, and some of those compounds are more concentrated in seeds, skins, and certain plant parts than in the softer edible flesh.

That's why preparation matters. If you use vegetables, favor lower-sugar options, keep portions modest, and choose preparation methods that may reduce digestive burden. This can include peeling, removing seeds when relevant, fermenting, or cooking thoroughly. This is especially important for people using vegetables as occasional tolerated extras rather than as major dietary staples. Zucchini, peeled cucumber, and asparagus are examples of vegetables that some people find easier to include because they're relatively low in digestible carbohydrate and less likely to take over the meal. Fermented vegetables such as kimchi or sauerkraut can also have a place, but mostly as condiments or small side portions rather than as major food groups. Fermented foods may support gut health for some people, but they aren't magic, and tolerance still matters.

Vegetable	Portion	Net Carbs	Preparation
Zucchini	1 medium	~4 g	Peel; cook thoroughly
Cucumber	½ cup	~2 g	Peel and de-seed
Asparagus	6 spears	~2 g	Steam or grill
Kimchi / Sauerkraut	¼ cup	varies	Fermented; watch additives

The Real Point of the Plant List

The purpose of this section isn't to encourage dietary drift. It's to create a controlled framework for the person who wants some flexibility without abandoning the advantages of an animal-based foundation. If adding avocado improves consistency without bringing cravings back, that may be useful. If a spoonful of sauerkraut makes meals more enjoyable and causes no problems, that may be useful. If berries quickly lead to more sweetness, more snacking, and a higher daily carb load, then they aren't useful, no matter how "healthy" they look on paper.

That's the real standard. Use plants only if they earn their place. They should add something without taking more than they give. If they increase cravings, destabilize appetite, worsen digestion, or quietly push the diet back toward old patterns, they don't belong in the protocol, no matter how socially acceptable they appear.

If you choose to include plants, let them enter as controlled variables, not emotional foods. Their job is to serve the framework, not slowly replace it.

The Sweetener Solution: Allulose as a Tactical Crutch

For many people, the hardest part of carnivore isn't meat, salt, or meal structure. It's sweetness. In the modern world, sugar isn't just a flavor. It's tied to reward, comfort, celebration, stress relief, and habit. When someone has spent years using sweet foods and drinks to get through the day, removing them can feel like more than a diet change. It can feel like withdrawal from a familiar emotional pattern. The palate does change for many people over time, but in the beginning, some people may need a controlled bridge instead of a purity contest.

This is where a tactical sweetener may have a place. The word tactical matters. The goal isn't to rebuild dessert culture with "approved" ingredients. The goal isn't to create a permanent dependence on sweet taste under a different label. The goal is to reduce the chance of a full relapse into junk food during the hardest part of the transition. If a small amount of a low-glycemic sweetener in coffee or tea helps someone avoid blowing up the entire protocol, that may be a reasonable short-term trade. The problem begins when the crutch quietly becomes a new habit.

WHAT IS ALLULOSE?

Allulose, also called D-allulose or D-psicose, is a rare sugar found naturally in very small amounts in foods such as figs and raisins. It's a monosaccharide, which means it's a simple sugar. Structurally, it's similar to fructose, but the body handles it differently. Unlike regular sugar, allulose contributes very few usable calories because most of it is absorbed and then excreted rather than fully metabolized for energy.

The strongest claim isn't that allulose has "zero insulin impact" in every person, in every dose, under every condition. The stronger claim is that allulose appears to have much smaller effects on blood sugar and insulin than regular sugar. Some research also suggests it may reduce the blood sugar rise that happens after eating carbohydrates, though that doesn't mean it should be used as an excuse to keep eating high-carb foods.

WHAT HAPPENS TO IT IN THE BODY?

A large portion of allulose is absorbed in the small intestine and then excreted in the urine instead of being fully used for energy. That's one reason it provides far fewer calories than regular sugar. In plain language, your body doesn't handle allulose the same way it handles table sugar.

This matters for carnivore because the practical concern isn't only calories. The bigger question is whether a sweetener brings back the blood sugar spikes and cravings that this way of eating is trying to remove. Allulose appears much less likely to raise blood sugar than regular sugar, but that doesn't automatically make it harmless from a behavior standpoint. A person can keep blood sugar stable while still feeding an attachment to sweet taste. Metabolic neutrality and behavioral neutrality aren't the same thing.

THE CRUTCH FACTOR

This is the part that matters most in real life. Allulose is best understood as a temporary tool, not a staple food. If someone is coming off a heavy dependence on sugar, sweetened coffee drinks, diet snacks, or evening desserts, a small amount of allulose may help reduce the odds of falling all the way back into processed food. But it should be used with the same caution as any crutch. A crutch is useful when it helps you get through a difficult phase. It becomes a problem when you never put it down.

That's why I'd keep its use narrow and intentional. Using a little in coffee or tea during the first few weeks is one thing. Rebuilding pancakes, cookies, sauces, and "carnivore desserts" around allulose is something else entirely. The more often sweetness is reintroduced, even in a lower-glycemic form, the more likely the palate stays trapped in the old pattern. The long-term aim of carnivore isn't just better blood sugar. It's a calmer relationship with food and less emotional dependence on sweetness.

THE PRACTICAL RULE

I used allulose during my own transition and found it genuinely useful for getting through the roughest weeks without blowing up the protocol entirely. That experience is part of why it's included here. But it's worth being honest about what allulose is and what it isn't. If you use it, use it sparingly and with a deadline. Treat it like nicotine gum for the sugar habit, not like a new permanent food group. Use the smallest amount necessary, avoid building rituals around it, and watch honestly for what it does to cravings.

If allulose helps you stay on plan without reactivating obsession, it may be useful. If it keeps the sweet tooth alive, it isn't helping, no matter how clever it looks. The real question isn't whether allulose is "allowed." The real question is whether it's moving you toward food freedom or simply giving sugar dependency a new costume.

Allulose can be a useful bridge, but bridges are meant to be crossed. If you stay on them too long, you never actually arrive. Also be aware that allulose can cause digestive distress, bloating, gas, or diarrhea when consumed in larger amounts. Start small. If another low-calorie sweetener works better for you and doesn't trigger cravings, that may be the better tool during transition.

THE TRAP OF "LOW-CARB" SUBSTITUTES

This is where many well-intentioned people stall. They remove sugar, bread, and junk food in name, but then rebuild the same eating pattern with "keto" labels. The package changes. The psychology stays the same. Instead of cookies, it becomes "keto cookies." Instead of tortillas, it becomes "low-carb tortillas." Instead of bread, it becomes "zero net carb bread." What looks like good keto food is often just the Standard American Diet wearing a low-carb costume.

That's why these products can be so dangerous. They let a person keep eating with the same rhythm, the same textures, the same emotional cues, and the same processed-food dependence while believing they have changed. But the whole point of a carnivore or strict animal-based framework isn't merely to lower carbohydrates. It's to simplify inputs, reduce food noise, and break the behavioral loop that keeps appetite, cravings, and decision-making unstable. Many processed low-carb substitutes work directly against that goal.

THE PROCESSED KETO PROBLEM

Walk down the "keto" aisle and look closely at the ingredient lists. Many of these products aren't built from food in any meaningful sense. They're food-like formulations. They're often held together with isolated fibers, wheat gluten, modified starches, gums, seed oils, and sweeteners designed to mimic familiar products while still qualifying for a marketing claim. In plain language, they're often engineered products designed to look like the old foods while pretending to be a clean replacement.

This matters because "low-carb" doesn't automatically mean low-impact. The net carb concept can be useful in some situations, but it isn't a guarantee of how a food will behave in your body. Blood sugar responses vary from person to person, and food-label shortcuts don't erase that biological reality. Two people can eat the same product and have very different post-meal glucose responses.

That doesn't mean every low-carb tortilla will spike everyone's glucose dramatically. The stronger and more accurate point is that the package math may not predict your real-world response as cleanly as the marketing suggests. A processed product can still interfere with appetite control, drive overeating, keep cravings alive, or produce a worse blood sugar response than expected, even if the label looks impressive.

THE BIGGER PROBLEM: PROCESSED FOOD BY ANOTHER NAME

Even if a low-carb substitute doesn't cause a big blood sugar response, it can still keep the old pattern alive. That's the deeper trap. A "keto brownie" may have less sugar than a regular brownie, but it still acts like dessert in the brain. It keeps the sweet taste front and center. It keeps the reward loop active. It keeps the brain expecting highly enjoyable processed food instead of learning to be satisfied with simpler meals. In that sense, the biggest problem with these foods is often behavioral, not just metabolic.

This is where many people quietly fail. They say they're eating low-carb, but they're still eating like snackers. They're still grazing, still chasing sweetness, still using packaged products as emotional food, and still relying on convenience formulas instead of real meals. The body may be getting less sugar, but the mind never gets the reset. The palate never changes. The craving loop never fully breaks.

There's another issue too, many of these products still belong in the category of ultra-processed foods. The argument isn't that every processed low-carb product is equally harmful. That would be too broad. The point is that rebuilding your diet around processed substitutes is moving in the wrong direction if the goal is metabolic stability, appetite control, and long-term health.

THE ONE-INGREDIENT RULE

That's why the one-ingredient rule is so useful. The closer your food stays to its original form, the less room there is for confusion, hidden additives, labeling tricks, and appetite manipulation.

Steak: ingredient - beef. Eggs: ingredient - eggs. Avocado: ingredient - avocado.

These foods don't require a paragraph of explanation, a net-carb loophole, or a marketing story to justify their place on your plate. They are food in a form your body can understand.

The one-ingredient rule doesn't mean every multi-ingredient food is automatically forbidden. It means complexity should have to earn its place. If a product needs a long ingredient list, a "net carb" defense, and an internet debate to explain why it's acceptable, then it's probably not helping you during transition.

THE PRACTICAL STANDARD

If your goal is healing, fat adaptation, appetite control, and a real reset in your relationship with food, then your standard must be stricter than the package label. Ask a better question than "Is this technically low-carb?" Ask, "Does this food simplify my system or complicate it?"

That's the standard.

If a product keeps you hungry, keeps you snacking, keeps you craving sweetness, keeps your gut unsettled, or keeps you mentally attached to the same processed food patterns you're trying to leave behind, then it isn't a tool. It's an obstacle.

Bottom Line

The low-carb substitute industry sells familiarity, not freedom. It gives people a way to keep eating processed food without forcing them to confront why processed food had so much power over them in the first place. Carnivore works best when it strips away that illusion. The closer you stay to recognizable, minimally processed foods, the faster the body and mind tend to calm down.

If a food has to be defended with label math, marketing language, and ingredient loopholes, it's probably not helping you move forward.

SUMMARY OF CHAPTER 6

In this chapter, we defined the ketovore bridge as a strategic tool, not a permanent destination. Its purpose isn't to rebuild the modern diet with cleaner branding. Its purpose is to provide a controlled layer of flexibility for people who need a more gradual path or who want limited variety without losing the animal-based foundation. The central lesson is that plant foods, sweeteners, and low-carb products should never be treated as automatic parts of the diet. They're optional variables, and their value depends entirely on whether they help preserve stability or quietly pull you backward.

We began by building a hierarchy of plant foods. Instead of treating all plants as equal, we ranked them according to how little trouble they're likely to cause. Fat-dominant fruits like avocado, olives, and unsweetened coconut were presented as the most useful bridge foods because they act more like fat sources than sugar sources. Low-sugar berries were framed as occasional garnish foods rather than staples, and lower-carbohydrate vegetables were treated with more caution, with an emphasis on modest portions and preparation methods that may reduce digestive burden. The broader rule wasn't ideological purity; it was carbohydrate control and careful experimentation. The plant list exists to support the framework, not to replace it.

We then examined allulose as a tactical crutch for people struggling with sweetness during transition. The chapter explained that allulose appears to have a much smaller blood sugar effect than regular sugar and may have some useful metabolic properties. But it also made clear that metabolic neutrality isn't the same as behavioral neutrality. A sweetener can avoid a major blood sugar spike and still keep the palate mentally attached to sweetness. That's why allulose was framed not as a staple, but as a temporary tool. It may help a person through the roughest phase of sugar withdrawal, but only if used sparingly and with the intention of letting it go.

Finally, we dismantled the trap of processed low-carb substitutes. "Keto" breads, tortillas, desserts, and snack products were exposed for what they often are, reformulations of the same processed-food mentality that carnivore is supposed to break. Even when carbohydrate counts look good on paper, these products often preserve the appetite patterns, psychology, and food complexity of the old system. The one-ingredient rule became the clearest defense against that trap. The closer food remains to its original form, the less room there is for ingredient games, metabolic surprises, and behavioral backsliding.

Chapter 7: The Soft Landing: 7-Day Transition Meal Plan

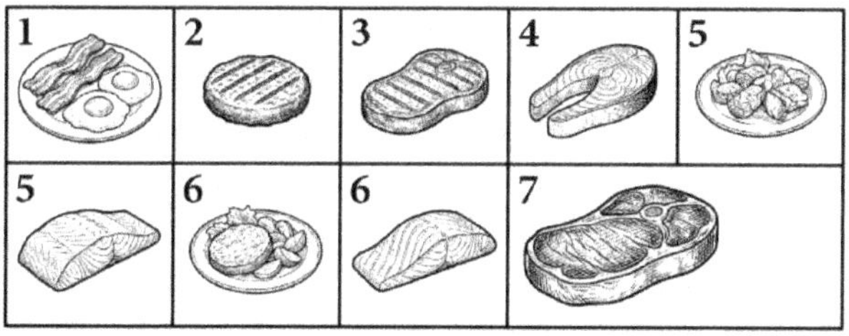

CHAPTER 7

THE SOFT LANDING, 7-DAY TRANSITION MEAL PLAN

Up to this point, we've covered the case for carnivore, the food hierarchy, the kitchen setup, the reality of adaptation, and the role of strategic flexibility. But knowledge by itself doesn't change behavior. It doesn't fill your plate, stop a craving, or help you make a better decision when you're tired, rushed, or hungry. Eventually, every dietary philosophy must work in real life. That's the purpose of this chapter.

This chapter is about action. It's where theory becomes food, and food becomes a plan. The Soft-Landing plan is designed to move you out of the high-carb instability of the modern diet and into a more stable animal-based rhythm without demanding perfection, calorie counting, or unnecessary complexity. It's built to reduce decision fatigue during the hardest part of the transition. Instead of asking yourself what to eat every time hunger shows up, you follow a clear framework for one week and let repetition do some of the work.

The reason this plan is called a soft landing is simple, not everyone does best by jumping straight from the modern diet into the strictest form of carnivore overnight. Some people do well starting hard and clean. Others do better with a more strategic step-down, one that keeps animal foods as the foundation while allowing a small amount of controlled flexibility, so the process doesn't collapse under early cravings, social pressure, or old habits. This plan reflects that reality. It blends stricter carnivore meals with selective ketovore flexibility, not to weaken the approach, but to make it more sustainable for someone still climbing out of the metabolic chaos of the standard diet.

The goal of this week isn't to impress anyone. It isn't to achieve perfect eating, prove toughness, or create the appearance of flawless discipline. The goal is to stabilize hunger, simplify decisions, reduce processed food exposure, and begin teaching the body what steady nourishment feels like. If the week goes well, you should come out of it with fewer cravings, better fullness, more confidence with meat-based meals, and a clearer sense of whether your body does best with stricter carnivore or benefits from a measured bridge.

How to Execute This Plan

Before you look at a single meal, you need to understand the operating rules for the week. These rules matter more than the exact menu because they determine how the plan is lived, not just how it's written.

- **The Satiety Rule**

Don't approach this week with a starvation mindset. This isn't the time to restrict aggressively, chase a calorie target, or prove how little food you can survive on. During transition, the body usually responds better to enough food than to strict under-eating. Eat until you're truly satisfied. "Thanksgiving full" may be colorful language, but the deeper principle is simple, you want the body to receive a clear signal that fuel is available. That helps reduce the sense of scarcity that often drives cravings, stress, and rebound eating.

If you're hungry again an hour after a meal, the first question shouldn't be, "How do I resist?" It should be, "Did I actually eat enough?" In many cases, the answer is no. Meals that are too lean or too small often set people up for failure later in the day. In the first week especially, satiety matters more than restraint.

- **The Snack Strategy**

Snacking isn't ideal, but strategic snacking is very different from chaotic snacking. If hunger shows up between meals, don't solve it with processed "keto" products, sweeteners, or convenience foods that keep the reward loop alive. Solve it with actual food. A hard-boiled egg, leftover burger patties, slices of cold steak, a few pieces of bacon, or another simple animal food will do far more for stability than a packaged low-carb product pretending to be helpful.

The purpose of the snack strategy isn't to create a grazing lifestyle. It's to prevent panic eating and poor decisions during a difficult transition phase. Use real food when needed, then return to structure.

- **The 2-Meal Evolution**

You'll notice that this plan often centers around two meals rather than three. That isn't because skipping breakfast is automatically better or because fasting is being forced on you. It's because when meals contain enough protein and fat, many people naturally find that hunger becomes less frequent and less urgent. Appetite often becomes calmer. Some people wake up and genuinely don't want breakfast. That's fine. Others still want a morning meal. That's also fine.

The plan is a guide, not a prison. If you're hungry, eat. If you're not hungry, don't force food out of habit. The point is to begin listening to real hunger signals instead of eating according to old patterns of blood sugar swings, convenience, boredom, or social conditioning.

- **The Simplicity Rule**

Don't overcomplicate this week. The transition works better when the food is simple, recognizable, and repeatable. That means plain meats, eggs if tolerated, animal fats, salt, and only limited bridge foods where the plan calls for them. Avoid the temptation to "upgrade" the plan with elaborate sauces, desserts, specialty products, or low-carb imitations of the foods you're trying to leave behind.

- **The Hydration and Salt Rule**

The first week is often when people feel changes in fluid and electrolyte balance most sharply. Keep fluids steady and salt your food generously. If you begin to feel foggy, crampy, weak, or unusually drained, don't automatically assume the plan is failing. It may simply mean you need more sodium, more water, or more total food. Sleep may also feel lighter or more broken during this week. That can happen during transition as the body adjusts to changes in fluid balance, minerals, and fuel use. Magnesium glycinate at night may help some people.

- **The Mindset Rule**

This week isn't about being perfect. It's about staying inside the framework long enough for the body to begin settling down. If one meal is imperfect, that isn't a reason to abandon the rest of the day. If social life forces an adjustment, make the best decision available and move on. Don't let one compromise become a full unraveling. Consistency beats theatrical perfection every time.

What This Plan Is Designed to Do

This 7-day plan has three jobs.

First, it lowers food noise. By reducing processed food, sugar, refined carbohydrates, and constant decision-making, it gives the body a cleaner signal.

Second, it increases satiety. Protein and fat are used on purpose because, when eaten in adequate amounts, they make the plan easier to sustain.

Third, it creates momentum. One good day helps. Seven structured days in a row can begin changing appetite, confidence, cravings, and meal habits in a way you can actually feel.

By the end of the week, you should know more than just what to eat. You should have a better sense of how your body responds to animal-based eating, how much food actually satisfies you, whether you need the bridge foods at all, and how much simpler life becomes when food stops being a constant negotiation.

The meals that follow aren't meant to be fancy. They're meant to work. Follow them honestly, eat enough, keep the food simple, and let the week teach you something.

The 7-Day Transition Plan

Day	**Meal 1** (Late Morning / Brunch)	**Meal 2** (Dinner)	**Notes:** Add a 3rd meal in there somewhere if needed. Plan to eat only when the sun is out. Unless you're a shift worker.
Mon	Classic Start: 4 eggs scrambled in generous butter, plus 4–6 slices of bacon	The Big Steak: 16 oz ribeye (reverse seared), topped with cold butter	Prioritize salt today. If a headache appears, add sea salt to water.

Tue	Leftovers: Cold sliced steak with 2 fried eggs (cooked in bacon grease, ghee, or butter)	Budget Bowl: 1 lb. ground beef (80/20) with shredded cheddar	Don't drain the fat, pour it over the meat.
Wed	Ketovore Lunch: 6 air-fried chicken wings with ½ avocado (salted)	Pork & Pickles: 2 pork chops (fried in tallow) with dill pickles (no sugar)	Avocado adds potassium to reduce early electrolyte symptoms.
Thur	Omelet: 3 eggs with chopped ham and Swiss cheese	Slow Cooker Feast: Chuck roast (8 hrs., salt and water), shredded	Save the broth, drink it as a salty electrolyte boost.
Fri	Fish Friday: Sardines (in water) or salmon, plus 2 hard-boiled eggs	Steak & "Dessert": NY strip steak with carnivore ice cream	Carnivore ice cream: blend heavy cream, egg yolks, and a small amount of allulose, then freeze. Optional. Allulose is discussed in Chapter 6.
Sat	The Scramble: Ground beef with 3 eggs and peeled zucchini slices	Lamb Night: Lamb chops or ground lamb patties	Lamb's fat profile often increases satiety.

Sun	The Compressed Window: Black coffee, or coffee with a small splash of heavy cream (optional allulose)	Sunday Roast: Brisket or prime rib, eaten until full	Black coffee alone is the cleanest version. Heavy cream makes it a "dirty fast" — useful for beginners, explained fully in Chapter 8.

YOUR FIRST WEEK SHOPPING LIST

To succeed, you need to remove the daily stress of asking, "What's for dinner?" Have these foods in your refrigerator, freezer, and pantry before Monday morning so the week starts with structure instead of guesswork.

The Meat Counter

- Ribeye or chuck steaks (2 lbs)
- 80/20 ground beef (3 lbs)
- Sugar-free bacon (2 packs)
- Chicken wings or thighs (1 pack)
- Pork chops (2 large)
- Chuck roast (3 to 4 lbs)
- Lamb chops or ground lamb (1 lb)
- Salmon, sardines, or another fatty fish (2 servings)

Dairy & Eggs

• Eggs (3 to 4 dozen)

• Grass-fed butter (1 lb)

• Heavy whipping cream (1 pint)

• Hard cheese, such as cheddar or Swiss (12 oz)

The Bridge - Optional

• Avocado (1)

• Zucchini (1)

• Dill pickles (12 oz), check for no added sugar or artificial dyes

Pantry Staples

• High-quality salt, such as Redmond Real Salt, Diamond Crystal kosher salt, Maldon salt flakes, or another mineral-rich salt (16 oz)

• Beef tallow or ghee (16 oz)

• Allulose, if using it as a temporary crutch (16 oz)

SUMMARY OF CHAPTER 7

Chapter 7 marks the shift from understanding the framework to actually living it. The 7-day Soft Landing plan isn't just a menu. It's a structured entry into the carnivore lifestyle designed to reduce decision fatigue, stabilize appetite, and make the first week more practical and less chaotic. Instead of leaving the transition to guesswork, this chapter gives you a clear system for your first seven days. It gives your body a simpler food environment and gives your mind fewer chances to drift.

The strength of this plan is its controlled flexibility. By combining stricter animal-based meals with carefully limited bridge foods, the chapter addresses some of the most common reasons people fail early, under-eating, poor meal structure, unmanaged cravings, and impulsive food choices when life gets inconvenient. The emphasis throughout the week isn't calorie counting, perfectionism, or diet theatrics. You learned that real food, not packaged low-carb substitutes, is what carries the transition. When meals are built around protein, fat, and enough total food, hunger often becomes calmer and easier to manage.

The chapter also reinforced several practical lessons that determine whether the first week feels stable or miserable. Fat was treated as fuel instead of something to fear, which is why meals were built to be satisfying rather than artificially lean. Simple snack options were included not to encourage grazing, but to prevent panic eating and poor decisions during vulnerable moments. Limited bridge foods were used strategically, not casually, to make the transition more manageable without rebuilding the old diet under a different label. The chapter also introduced the idea that many people naturally begin to shorten their eating window once satiety improves, not because fasting is being forced, but because appetite often becomes less constant when blood sugar swings and processed foods are reduced.

Most importantly, this week was designed to create momentum. By the end of the seven days, the goal wasn't perfection, but proof. Proof that meals can be simpler. Proof that cravings can begin to quiet down. Proof that the body may respond well to an animal-based rhythm when it's given enough food and fewer mixed signals. That's the real purpose of the Soft Landing.

Chapter 8: Intermittent Fasting: The Force Multiplier

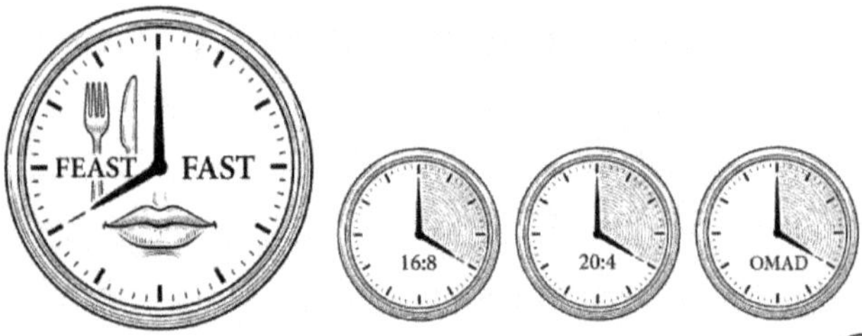

CHAPTER 8

INTERMITTENT FASTING: THE FORCE MULTIPLIER

Intermittent fasting is often presented as a test of discipline, but in a properly built carnivore framework, it's better understood as a secondary tool that becomes available once the food itself is doing its job. When meals are built around enough protein, enough fat, and enough total food, hunger often becomes quieter, steadier, and less demanding. In that environment, going longer between meals can begin to feel natural instead of punishing. That's when fasting becomes useful, not as an act of force, but as an extension of metabolic stability.

This chapter approaches intermittent fasting from that perspective. It isn't a diet, and it isn't a moral achievement. It's a meal-timing strategy. It doesn't decide what belongs on the plate, earlier chapters already established that. What it changes is the spacing between meals. That spacing can affect appetite, insulin exposure, daily structure, and, in some cases, how easily the body uses stored fuel. Fasting works best when it's built on a stable nutritional foundation. If the diet is still chaotic, if hunger is still unpredictable, if the body is underfed and overstressed, or if sleep is consistently poor, fasting can become another stressor instead of a force multiplier.

That's why carnivore and intermittent fasting can work well together, but they shouldn't be treated as automatic partners. Carnivore often makes fasting easier because satiety improves and cravings lose some of their urgency. At the same time, fasting isn't better just because it's difficult, and it isn't required for success. Some people do well with a simple 12:12 schedule, meaning 12 hours of fasting and a 12-hour eating window. Others do well with 16:8, meaning 16 hours of fasting and an 8-hour eating window. Others do better avoiding aggressive fasting until recovery, hormones, training, sleep, and appetite are more stable. The goal isn't to worship fasting. The goal is to understand when it helps, when it hurts, and how to use it without turning it into another form of dietary chaos.

Navigating the Fasting Landscape

Fasting is a tool, not a moral achievement. It can be useful, but its value depends on context, your metabolic health, your stress load, your activity level, your relationship with food, and whether fasting helps you become more stable or simply makes you more obsessive. Too many people treat fasting like a religion. They assume longer is always better, harder is always cleaner, and hunger is always proof of progress. That thinking is sloppy. Fasting only works when it serves the body instead of becoming another form of self-imposed chaos.

In the carnivore framework, fasting often becomes easier because satiety improves. When meals are built around enough protein and fat, hunger tends to feel less erratic and less urgent than it does on a carbohydrate-heavy diet. That doesn't mean everyone should immediately start skipping meals. It means fasting should come from improved appetite control. If you're white-knuckling your way through a fasting window while under-eating, craving constantly, and feeling depleted, you aren't practicing advanced discipline. You're probably just undernourished.

The first principle is simple, earn the right to fast. Before you experiment with shorter eating windows or longer fasts, you should already be eating real food consistently, getting enough electrolytes, recovering well, and experiencing reasonably stable hunger. Fasting works best when it's built on top of nutritional stability, not when it's used to compensate for a broken food pattern. Research suggests that intermittent fasting and time-restricted eating may help with weight loss and some metabolic markers in people who are overweight or obese, but the results depend heavily on adherence, the specific fasting schedule, and the person's overall context.

A Practical Fasting Hierarchy

- **12:12 — Fast 12 Hours, Eat 12 Hours**

  Difficulty: Very easy.

This is the true entry point, even if people rarely get excited about it. A 12:12 schedule is basically a structured overnight fast with a clear eating window. It's often the best place to start because it creates rhythm without creating unnecessary stress. For someone coming off constant snacking, late-night eating, and unstable hunger, simply closing the kitchen at night and eating again the next morning at a reasonable hour can be a meaningful step.

This teaches the body that food doesn't need to be available around the clock. It also supports a better daily rhythm, which matters more than most people realize. The goal isn't to prove toughness. The goal is to create structure.

Best for: beginners, people with a long snacking history, and those who need structure before they need ambition.

- **16:8 — Fast 16 Hours, Eat 8 Hours**

  Difficulty: Easy.

This is the most popular version of intermittent fasting for a reason, it's simple, realistic, and often sustainable. For many people, especially once carnivore improves satiety, a 16:8 pattern begins to happen naturally. Breakfast becomes optional, lunch and dinner become more substantial, and the constant pull toward food starts to quiet down.

This schedule is often the sweet spot for many adults because it provides a meaningful fasting period without pushing too far into recovery problems, social interference, or unnecessary rigidity. Time-restricted eating may help improve body weight, waist size, and some metabolic markers for some people, but it isn't automatically better than simply eating less overall. The benefit depends on the person, the food quality, and whether the schedule is actually sustainable.

Best for: most people who already have better satiety and want more structure.

- **20:4 —Fast 20 Hours, Eat 4 Hours - The Warrior Way**

Difficulty: Moderate.

A 20:4 schedule compresses eating into a narrow window. For most people, that usually means one large meal plus a smaller follow-up meal, or two meals eaten close together. This can work well for some busy people because it simplifies the day and reduces the number of food decisions.

A narrow window can be useful if it helps you stay focused and still allows you to eat enough. But it can backfire if the compressed schedule turns into chronic under-eating, rushed meals, poor training recovery, or a daily cycle of deprivation followed by overeating. The body may tolerate a 20:4 pattern well if total food intake stays high enough. It may also read it as scarcity if the execution is poor. That distinction matters more than the fasting window itself.

Best for: experienced people with stable hunger, busy schedules, and enough appetite to eat properly in a short window.

- **OMAD — One Meal a Day**

  Difficulty: Hard.

OMAD has a certain psychological appeal because it feels clean, disciplined, and extreme in a way that many people find attractive. But it isn't automatically better, and it's often less appropriate than its reputation suggests. Eating once a day can work for some experienced carnivores whose appetite is truly calm and who can comfortably eat enough food in one sitting. It can also become a disguised form of chronic underfeeding.

This is especially important for people who train hard, who are still adapting, who have a history of restriction, or who do poorly with huge meals. OMAD isn't a sign of advanced metabolism if it leaves you cold, irritable, under-recovered, or obsessed with food. More extreme fasting isn't automatically more effective. The benefit is usually context-specific, not simply a matter of longer being better.

Best for: experienced carnivores with strong satiety, stable energy, and no signs of under-recovery.

- **ADF — Alternate-Day Fasting**
  Difficulty: Hard.

Alternate-day fasting is one of the more aggressive tools in the fasting world. It usually means either a full 36-hour fast or a major calorie reduction every other day. It can help some people lose weight and improve certain metabolic markers, but it's much harder to sustain than simpler fasting schedules. Long-term consistency is the real problem. A fasting plan that looks powerful on paper but creates rebound eating, stress, or obsession isn't a good plan.

This isn't where beginners should start. Alternate-day fasting is better treated as a situational tool for people who are already stable, already adapted, and using it deliberately instead of emotionally. It may have a place for some people dealing with a stubborn plateau, but it also comes with a larger recovery cost and a higher risk of overeating afterward if the basic food pattern isn't already solid.

Best for: selected cases, experienced fasters, and plateaus approached strategically rather than emotionally.

There are even more aggressive fasting schedules not discussed in this book.

How to Choose the Right Protocol

The correct protocol is the least aggressive one that gives you the benefit you need. That's the real rule. If 12:12 or 16:8 improves appetite control, simplifies your day, and supports steady progress, then there's no prize for escalating to OMAD. If OMAD leaves you depleted, irritable, cold, under-recovered, or obsessed with food, you aren't failing by stepping back. You're making a smarter adjustment.

Meal timing also matters. Fasting shouldn't be viewed only as a contest of how long you can avoid food. The body runs on rhythm. For many people, eating earlier in the day and avoiding large late-night meals works better than saving most of the food for the evening. That doesn't mean everyone has to eat early, but it does mean fasting should respect circadian rhythm, sleep, digestion, and recovery.

When Not to Push Fasting Harder

This is where maturity matters. Fasting is a poor tool to escalate when you're newly transitioning, under-eating, sleeping poorly, training heavily, struggling with binge tendencies, dealing with hormone problems, or showing signs of low energy availability. Sleep deprivation especially works against the hormonal environment fasting is supposed to support. In those situations, longer fasting is often the wrong move. It may produce short-term scale movement while quietly making the real problem worse.

Women, especially those with signs of low energy availability or cycle changes, should be careful about turning fasting into a daily stressor. People with diabetes, people taking glucose-lowering medication, pregnant or breastfeeding women, people with a history of eating disorders, and people with complex medical conditions need extra caution. Fasting can interact with medications, blood sugar regulation, hormones, and recovery in ways that aren't minor.

The Deeper Purpose of Fasting

The real purpose of fasting isn't suffering. Fasting can simplify life, improve meal structure, reduce mindless eating, and, in some cases, support metabolic health. But once fasting becomes a performance identity, it usually stops being useful. The best fasting protocol is the one that makes your life calmer, your appetite steadier, and your recovery more reliable. Anything beyond that is often ego wearing a health costume.

Protocol	Schedule	Best For	Difficulty
12:12	Fast 12h / Eat 12h (e.g., 8am–8pm)	Beginners	Very easy
16:8	Fast 16h / Eat 8h	Most individuals	Easy

20:4 (Warrior)	Fast 20h / Eat 4h	Busy professionals	Moderate
OMAD	One meal daily	Experienced carnivores	Hard
ADF	Alternate-day fasting (36h fast)	Plateaus	Hard

Why Skip a Meal? The Science of Scarcity

Human physiology wasn't built around constant feeding. Food was once intermittent, not available all day, every day. Our ancestors didn't wake up to a kitchen full of options, snack through the afternoon, and go to bed while digestion was still working overtime. They had periods of eating and periods without food, and the body developed ways to function in both states. That doesn't mean every modern person should fast aggressively. It means the body is capable of handling time without food, and in some cases, that time may create useful biological effects.

The value of fasting isn't that it makes you suffer. The value is that it creates a different internal environment than constant eating.

This distinction matters because modern life normalizes nonstop intake. Many people go from coffee to breakfast, from breakfast to snacks, from snacks to lunch, from lunch to "healthy" treats, and from dinner to dessert without giving digestion, insulin, or appetite signals much time to quiet down. Fasting reintroduces that quiet. It creates a period where the body is no longer focused on incoming food and can shift more attention toward using stored fuel, improving metabolic flexibility, and maintaining internal systems. The effects aren't magic, and they aren't the same for every person, but the basic principle is sound, time without food changes what the body is doing.

AUTOPHAGY: THE CELLULAR HOUSECLEANING

Autophagy is one of the most talked-about parts of fasting, and one of the most exaggerated. At its core, autophagy is a normal cellular cleanup process. The body breaks down and recycles damaged proteins, worn-out cell parts, and other internal waste. It isn't the body "eating itself" in some scary way. It's basic maintenance, repair, and quality control.

Fasting can support autophagy-related pathways, but the timing isn't as simple as internet fasting culture makes it sound. It would be too strong to say that autophagy automatically "starts" or "ramps up" at one exact hour for every person. The safer and more accurate point is this; going without food is one of the stresses that can encourage cellular cleanup and recycling, and longer periods without food may increase that signal more than constant eating. But the exact timing varies by person, activity level, metabolic state, and overall context.

The practical takeaway is still useful. By creating time away from constant food intake, fasting may allow the body to spend more time in maintenance and recycling mode instead of always processing incoming food. That's one reason fasting is interesting beyond weight loss. It shifts the body's internal message from "process and store what's coming in" to "use, repair, recycle, and reorganize what's already here."

RESTORING INSULIN SENSITIVITY

Every time you eat, insulin rises to some degree. That's normal. Insulin isn't the enemy. The problem is when the body is exposed to too much food too often for too long, especially in the context of poor food quality, excess body fat, poor sleep, and low activity. Over time, the system can become less responsive. Fasting can help by increasing the time between insulin rises and giving the body more time to use stored fuel instead of constantly processing incoming food.

That said, fasting isn't the only way to improve insulin sensitivity, and it isn't automatically better than every other tool. Better food quality, lower carbohydrate intake, weight loss, better sleep, and more movement can all matter just as much, and sometimes more, depending on the person. The stronger claim is that fasting can be one useful way to reduce feeding frequency and improve metabolic flexibility. It isn't the only lever that matters.

Within a carnivore framework, this often becomes easier because meals built around protein and fat tend to keep people satisfied longer. That means fasting may begin to happen naturally instead of being forced. A person who's no longer trapped in constant cravings and blood sugar swings may find that skipping a meal feels less like deprivation and more like a normal extension of being satisfied. That's the best context for fasting, not as punishment, but as a byproduct of stability.

Cognitive Clarity and Signal Restoration

One of the most common things people report during fasting is better mental clarity. Many describe a quieter mind, sharper focus, or a more alert feeling when they aren't digesting food. There are possible reasons for this, including steadier energy availability and ketone use, but the experience isn't identical for everyone.

Many people in fasting and carnivore communities describe this state as "predatory focus." They mean a sense of sharper alertness and less mental noise that can happen when digestion is quiet and the brain feels like it's running on cleaner fuel. That phrase captures something real for many people, but it should be treated as a personal description, not a scientific guarantee. Some people feel mentally sharper when fasted. Others feel distracted, irritable, weak, or underpowered, especially if they're under-slept, underfed, overstressed, or still adapting.

Still, the broader point is useful. Digestion takes energy. When you aren't eating, the body is operating in a different mode, and for some people that mode feels cleaner, more alert, and less noisy. In a world where constant eating is normal, that contrast can feel powerful. Whether you explain it through ketones, reduced digestive demand, or simply a break from the constant rhythm of eating, the experience is one reason many people keep fasting as a tool.

The Real Reason to Skip a Meal

A well-timed fast can simplify the day, reduce mindless eating, reinforce satiety signals, and give the body a stretch of time when it isn't processing incoming food. That may support metabolic health, and it may create real benefits in energy and focus for some people. But fasting should be treated as a controlled stressor, not a moral badge. The person who skips a meal because he's genuinely not hungry is in a very different place from the person who skips a meal because he's trying to punish his body into submission.

The bottom line is simple, measured scarcity can activate processes that constant abundance may suppress. But those effects aren't all-or-nothing, and they don't justify turning fasting into mythology. Skip a meal when it serves the system. Don't skip one just because suffering makes the practice feel more serious.

How to Fast on Carnivore: The Intuitive Way

The most common fasting mistake is trying to force a schedule before the body is stable enough to handle it. On carnivore, fasting works best when it grows out of satiety. If you're still dealing with strong sugar cravings, getting shaky or irritable between meals, or thinking about food constantly, you usually aren't ready to push fasting harder. Forcing a fasting protocol too early often backfires because the body isn't yet calm enough to support it.

This is why the intuitive approach matters. Start by building meals that are actually satisfying. In practice, that usually means eating real meals built around enough protein and enough fat, while reducing snacks where possible. Once satiety improves, many people naturally begin stretching the time between meals without staring at a clock. Breakfast becomes optional instead of mandatory. The eating window narrows because appetite has calmed down. Some people naturally settle into something like a 16:8 rhythm, but that should be treated as a possible outcome, not a deadline or a requirement.

A practical progression looks like this. First, eat consistently enough that blood sugar swings and panic hunger begin to fade. Second, make meals satisfying enough that you aren't hunting for snacks an hour later. Third, let the first skipped meal happen naturally rather than ceremonially. That's the turning point. A person who forgets breakfast because he's truly not hungry is in a different physical and mental place than a person who skips breakfast while obsessing over lunch. The first is moving toward stability. The second is usually still negotiating with deprivation.

CLEAN VS. DIRTY FASTING

The language of "clean" and "dirty" fasting is useful as shorthand, but it shouldn't become dogma. The science isn't neat enough for that. A clean fast usually means water, salt, electrolytes and maybe plain tea and black coffee. The reasoning is simple; these provide little or no energy and are less likely to interrupt the fasting state than foods or drinks that contain calories.

That's why I wouldn't claim that a clean fast automatically "maximizes autophagy" as if that has been perfectly mapped in real humans. The safer and stronger claim is this, if your goal is to keep the fast as clear and simple as possible, plain fluids and salt make the most sense. They keep the fasting period cleaner than cream, broth, or other calorie-containing additions.

A "dirty" fast is best understood as a fast that includes a small calorie assist, such as a splash of heavy cream in coffee or a cup of bone broth. Those additions may make fasting easier mentally, and they may still allow someone to stay low-carb or ketogenic depending on the rest of the diet. But once calories enter, the fast is no longer the same as water, coffee, tea, and salt alone. It may still be useful. It's just not the cleanest version of the tool.

If black coffee and water are easy for you, keep the fast simple. If a small amount of cream genuinely helps you avoid blowing up the entire day with a pastry or a binge, then that may be a reasonable transition compromise. But call it what it is, a compromise that supports consistency, not a loophole that preserves every benefit of a stricter fast. The hierarchy still matters. Water, salt, tea, and black coffee are the cleaner options. Small calorie additions are the more forgiving option. Neither should be turned into a religion.

What Matters Most

The real question isn't whether your fast is pure enough to impress internet fasting culture. The real question is whether fasting is making your life better. Is food taking up less mental space? Are you less reactive around food? Are you less dependent on constant intake? If the answer is yes, the tool is doing its job. If fasting makes you more obsessive, more depleted, or more likely to rebound into chaotic eating, then the protocol is wrong for your current state, no matter how "clean" it looks on paper.

When Fasting Goes Wrong: Recognizing Overload

Fasting can be a useful stressor, but useful stress only remains useful when the body can recover from it. That's the basic idea behind hormesis, the right dose of stress can make the system stronger, but too much stress becomes damaging.

Fasting is no different. In the right context, it can improve structure, reduce mindless eating, and support metabolic flexibility. In the wrong context, especially when stacked on top of poor sleep, psychological stress, hard training, and not enough food, it can become one more signal of scarcity in a body that's already stretched too thin.

This is where many people get into trouble. They assume that because fasting can be helpful, more fasting must be more helpful. That logic breaks down quickly in real life. A body that's sleeping poorly, working a high-stress job, training hard, and under-eating may not interpret longer fasting as a smart health tool. It may interpret it as cumulative stress. This is especially important for women because low energy availability can disrupt reproductive and hormone function, especially when food restriction and training stress are stacked together.

THE WARNING SIGNS

The warning signs of overload usually aren't subtle if you're willing to look at them honestly. Feeling cold all the time, persistent fatigue, irritability, declining workout performance, poor recovery, sleep disruption, hair thinning, low sex drive, and, in women, cycle changes or loss of a period can all suggest that the body is no longer reading fasting as a useful challenge. It may be reading it as a threat.

These symptoms aren't specific to fasting alone. They can also reflect other issues such as thyroid problems, low energy availability, illness, undernutrition, or broader hormone disruption. That's exactly why they shouldn't be romanticized or ignored. Feeling cold all the time, losing hair, sleeping poorly, and losing a menstrual cycle aren't badges of discipline. They're warning lights.

For women, this deserves special emphasis. Menstrual irregularity isn't a sign that the diet is "working harder." It's a sign that the reproductive system may be downshifting because the body doesn't feel adequately fueled or recovered.

THE CORRECTION

When these signs appear, the answer isn't more force. The answer is more support. Shorten the fasting window. Increase total food intake. Make sure meals are actually large enough and nourishing enough to restore energy. On a carnivore framework, that often means increasing dietary fat and avoiding the mistake of trying to live on lean protein while training hard and fasting aggressively. The body is more likely to recover, perform, and use stored fuel well when total stress is manageable and food intake is adequate. It doesn't work better when every variable is pushing toward scarcity at the same time.

Sleep also belongs in the correction. Fasting on top of poor sleep is one of the fastest ways to turn a useful tool into a net negative. Poor sleep makes appetite harder to control, lowers stress tolerance, weakens recovery, and makes the entire system more fragile. If fasting is making sleep worse, recovery worse, and hunger more chaotic, then fasting isn't helping. It's adding stress to an already stressed system.

THE PRACTICAL RULE

The practical rule is simple, if fasting makes you feel calmer, steadier, and less obsessed with food, it may be serving you. If it makes you chronically cold, depleted, hormonally unstable, or mentally brittle, it isn't. Don't confuse the ability to endure stress with the ability to benefit from it. Those aren't the same thing. The body adapts well only when stress is matched with recovery.

TROUBLESHOOTING COMMON ISSUES & PLATEAUS

The road to metabolic freedom is rarely linear. Progress doesn't move in a neat downward line, and the body doesn't always reward good decisions on your preferred timeline. That's why plateaus create so much frustration. People expect the system to respond like a machine. Instead, it responds like biology, unevenly, adaptively, and sometimes with delays that test patience more than discipline. A stall doesn't automatically mean the plan has failed. More often, it means something in the system needs to be interpreted more honestly.

This is the first principle of troubleshooting, don't confuse a pause with defeat. Weight can stall because of water retention, stress, poor sleep, hormone changes, digestive contents, inconsistent adherence, reduced daily movement, metabolic adaptation, or the simple fact that fat loss doesn't always show up on the scale in a straight line.

THE WEIGHT-LOSS STALL

If the scale hasn't moved in weeks, the first mistake is usually panic. The second mistake is trying to solve that panic with more aggression, more fasting, more restriction, more cardio, more punishment. Sometimes that works briefly. Often, it just adds more stress to a system that may already be pressing the brakes. Poor sleep and chronic stress aren't minor details. They can affect appetite, recovery, food choices, water retention, and weight regulation.

That's why a stall should trigger a review, not an emotional reaction. Ask better questions. How have you been sleeping? Has life stress increased? Are you training harder than usual and recovering worse? Have your meal sizes quietly shrunk because your appetite improved but your total food intake became too low? Are you weighing yourself at inconsistent times? Are you constipated, sore, inflamed, or holding water from travel, poor sleep, or a hard training block? Those questions matter more than the impulse to punish yourself with stricter fasting just because the scale offended you.

Sometimes the correct response to a stall isn't less food. Sometimes it's more stability. Better sleep. Lower stress. More consistent meals. A temporary return to two large, satisfying meals instead of a more aggressive fasting schedule. That doesn't mean stress explains every plateau. That would be too simple. It means sleep, stress, and recovery should be checked before you declare the diet broken.

There's also a harder truth people often resist, sometimes the plateau isn't a physiological mystery. Sometimes it's drift. Portions get sloppy. Bridge foods become frequent. Dairy creeps up. Low-carb processed keto products sneak in. Weekend exceptions turn into weekly patterns. The system stops being clean enough to deliver clear feedback.

LOW ENERGY

If you still feel sluggish weeks into the diet, don't assume the answer is more toughness. Low energy can come from several places. Early adaptation itself can cause fatigue, weakness, and a heavy feeling while the body adjusts to a different fuel system. This is especially true when sodium, fluids, fat, and total food intake aren't handled well.

But if low energy continues beyond the early transition, one of the first suspects is under-eating, especially under-eating fat. Many people say they're eating carnivore while still trying to hold on to a low-fat mindset. The result is predictable, meals are too lean, satisfaction is weak, energy is unstable, and the person feels like the system is running on fumes. If your meat looks dry, if your meals feel "clean" but not satisfying, or if you're hungry again too soon, the issue may not be a lack of protein. It may be that you're still starving the fuel side of the equation.

That doesn't mean every low-energy episode is fixed by adding butter to everything. It means fat intake, sodium, hydration, and total food should all be reviewed before you assume the diet itself is flawed. If the system feels underpowered, the first question should be whether you're actually giving it enough energy to run.

THE PLATEAU MINDSET

The mature way to troubleshoot is to stop treating every problem like a final judgment on the diet. A plateau isn't always sabotage. Low energy isn't always a deficiency. Social pressure isn't always proof that you're doing something wrong. Sometimes the issue is execution. Sometimes it's an adaptation. Sometimes it's stress. Sometimes it's simple impatience.

The right sequence is this, simplify, review, adjust, then wait. Clean up drift. Recheck sleep. Recheck stress.

Recheck sodium, hydration, fat, and total food. Recheck whether the diet is still as clean as you claim it is. Then give the body enough time to respond before creating a new problem through overreaction.

SUMMARY OF CHAPTER 8

In this chapter, we shifted from the question of what to eat to the question of when to eat. Intermittent fasting wasn't presented as a badge of discipline or a shortcut for suffering. It was presented as a tool that may become useful once hunger is more stable and meals are nourishing enough. The central lesson was that fasting works best when it grows out of satiety and structure, not force. A person who's eating enough protein and fat, experiencing calmer appetite, and no longer trapped in constant cravings is in a far better position to use fasting intelligently than someone still trying to white-knuckle his way through the day. Research on intermittent fasting suggests that the benefits can be real, but they depend heavily on context, consistency, the specific protocol, and overall food quality.

We also examined the biology behind fasting with more precision. Fasting can create a different internal environment than constant eating. It may support better insulin sensitivity, greater use of stored fuel, and cellular maintenance processes such as autophagy-related signaling. At the same time, the chapter made clear that these mechanisms are often exaggerated in popular culture, especially when exact timelines are presented as settled fact. The more honest conclusion is that fasting changes what the body is doing in meaningful ways, but the size and timing of those effects vary by person and are still being studied, especially in humans.

From there, we established the importance of intuitive fasting. You learned that the smartest progression isn't to force an aggressive schedule too early, but to let fasting windows narrow naturally as satiety improves. A 12:12 or 16:8 rhythm may be enough for many people, while more aggressive protocols such as 20:4, OMAD, or alternate-day fasting should be treated as optional tools rather than default goals. We also clarified the difference between "clean" and "dirty" fasting, not as a moral divide, but as a practical one. Water, black coffee, tea, and salt create the clearest fasting conditions, while small calorie additions may be useful transition compromises if they improve consistency, even though they no longer represent the same physiological state as a stricter fast.

Finally, the chapter addressed the reality that progress is rarely linear. Weight-loss stalls and low energy were reframed not as reasons to abandon the process, but as signals to review execution more honestly. Sometimes the problem is stress, poor sleep, under-eating, or hidden dietary drift. Sometimes the issue is social pressure rather than biology. The broader lesson was that consistency matters more than drama. With a better understanding of fasting, appetite, adaptation, and troubleshooting, you're no longer using meal timing as a gimmick. You're learning how to use it as leverage.

Chapter 9: The Probiotic Boost (Fermented Foods)

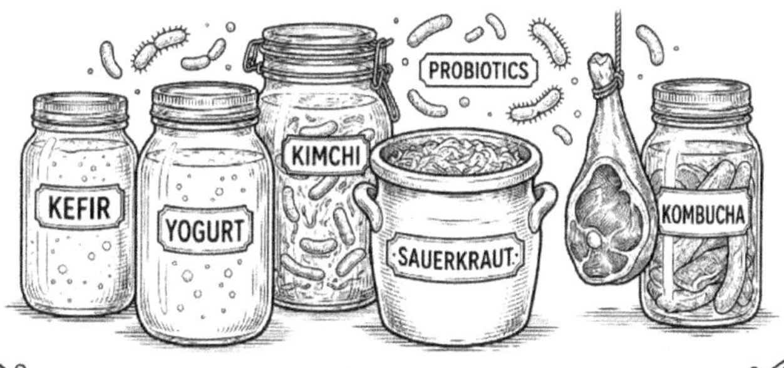

CHAPTER 9

THE PROBIOTIC BOOST, FERMENTED FOODS

While a strict Lion Diet of ruminant meat, salt, and water is the clearest elimination approach, many people find that carefully chosen fermented foods can help with long-term sustainability and digestion. Within the ketovore framework, these foods can act as a bridge between the simplicity of carnivore and the more complex needs of the gut.

Fermentation is one of the oldest food technologies humans ever used. Long before refrigeration, people used salt, time, and bacteria to preserve food. During fermentation, microbes consume some of the sugars in the food and can change certain plant compounds, making the food easier for some people to tolerate. In simple terms, fermentation partially breaks food down before you eat it. That doesn't make fermented foods magic, and it doesn't mean everyone needs them. But for people adjusting their digestion during a dietary transition, fermented foods may offer a small layer of support if they're used strategically and judged honestly by results.

Keep in mind that if store bought fermented items are not your thing due to the crappy ingredients, you can easily make you own.

Animal-Based Ferments: The Synergistic Choice

For people who tolerate dairy well, fermented dairy can be one of the more logical additions to a ketovore, or carnivore-adjacent framework. The reason is simple, these foods keep much of the protein, fat, and mineral value of dairy while fermentation changes the food in ways that may make it easier to tolerate for some people. That doesn't make fermented dairy mandatory, and it doesn't make it universally beneficial. It simply means it can be considered as an optional tool rather than an automatic staple.

This is where animal-based ferments differ from many plant ferments. They don't come with a large fiber load, and for some people, that makes them easier to fit into a lower-residue, animal-based diet. The advantage isn't that they're magically better than every other fermented food.

The advantage is that they may provide live cultures, fermentation byproducts, protein, and fat in a form that fits more naturally into a carnivore-leaning approach than large servings of fermented vegetables or plant-heavy probiotic foods.

That still depends on dairy tolerance. If dairy triggers congestion, skin problems, bloating, cravings, or stalled progress, fermentation doesn't automatically solve the problem. Fermented dairy is still dairy. It may be easier for some people, but it isn't a free pass.

THE POWER OF KEFIR

Kefir is one of the more interesting fermented dairy foods because it's usually made with a mixed culture of bacteria and yeasts, not just one or two starter organisms. That makes kefir more complex than standard yogurt and is one reason it has received attention in gut and metabolic health discussions.

Its most practical benefit isn't that it "kills bad bacteria" in some simplistic way. A better way to say it is that kefir may help influence the gut environment through live cultures, fermentation byproducts, and changes in gut signaling. Some people also tolerate kefir better than regular milk because fermentation can reduce lactose and make the dairy easier to handle. That makes kefir potentially useful for some people who tolerate dairy but don't do well with plain milk.

That said, kefir claims are easy to exaggerate. It's better to say that kefir may support gut health, lactose tolerance, and certain metabolic markers in some people than to present it as a guaranteed fix for gut problems. The evidence is promising in places, but it isn't strong enough to justify miracle language.

Selection matters. Unsweetened kefir is the version that makes the most sense in this framework. Added sugar defeats much of the point. Full-fat kefir usually fits better into an animal-based diet than low-fat kefir because it's more satisfying and keeps the food closer to its natural form.

Dose matters too. Kefir is usually better treated as an accent, not something to drink by the glass all day. A small serving with or after a meat-heavy meal may be enough to test tolerance without turning it into a major carbohydrate source. The goal isn't to replace meat with kefir. The goal is to see whether a modest amount of fermented dairy adds anything useful without creating problems.

Greek Yogurt

Greek yogurt, or strained yogurt, has a different role. Because it's strained, some of the whey is removed. This concentrates the protein and usually lowers lactose and carbohydrates compared with regular yogurt. That's one reason Greek yogurt can be easier to fit into a lower-carbohydrate framework.

Its main practical value is simplicity. It can provide a dense protein source, a thick texture, and live cultures in a form that some people tolerate better than milk. It isn't necessary, and it isn't automatically gentle on every gut. I wouldn't claim that it heals the intestinal lining in any direct or guaranteed way. The cleaner statement is this, some people find plain, unsweetened Greek yogurt easier to digest than milk and useful as a high-protein fermented dairy option.

The label rule should be strict. Milk and live cultures should be the baseline. Once you start seeing thickeners, starches, gums, sweeteners, or "natural flavors," the product is moving away from what makes it useful in the first place. This matters even more in a ketovore framework, where the value of a food often depends on how few unnecessary variables it brings into the system.

HOW TO USE FERMENTED DAIRY INTELLIGENTLY

The best way to think about animal-based ferments is as optional tools, not foundational foods. Meat remains the base. Fermented dairy, if tolerated, may add variety, a different texture, and potentially useful microbial activity. But the burden of proof stays on the food. If kefir or Greek yogurt improves consistency, causes no digestive problems, doesn't trigger skin or sinus issues, and doesn't reignite cravings, it may have a place. If it brings back congestion, acne, bloating, cravings, or stalled fat loss, then its theoretical benefits don't matter for your body.

That's the rule that keeps this section honest. Fermented dairy may be useful. It isn't automatically useful. Test it the same way you'd test any other gray-area food, by results, not by reputation.

PLANT-BASED FERMENTS

If plant foods are going to enter a ketovore framework, fermented vegetables make more sense than most other options. Fermentation can change plant chemistry, reduce some irritating compounds, create organic acids, and turn the food into something different from its raw form. That doesn't make fermented vegetables harmless for everyone, and it doesn't mean every plant suddenly becomes "safe" once fermented. But it can make certain vegetables more workable as small, strategic additions than they would be raw or heavily processed.

That's why these foods should be treated as condiments, not staples. Their role isn't to rebuild a vegetable-heavy diet. Their role is to offer flavor, acidity, and possibly some fermented-food benefits in a very small amount. The smaller the serving, the less likely it is to disrupt the animal-based foundation. If a spoonful improves consistency or meal enjoyment without creating cravings, bloating, or carb drift, it may have a place. If it turns into a bowlful, it has already stopped acting like a condiment.

Sauerkraut: The Fermented Cabbage Option

True sauerkraut is one of the simplest fermented vegetables, cabbage, salt, and time. During fermentation, lactic acid bacteria change the cabbage and create a sour, acidic environment that helps preserve the food. If the sauerkraut is unpasteurized, it may also contain live organisms and fermentation byproducts that can influence the gut environment.

The strongest claim here isn't that sauerkraut is a miracle digestive aid. The stronger claim is that fermented cabbage may provide useful microbial and fermentation-related signals in a small serving, and some people find it helpful for digestion. That doesn't mean everyone needs it, and it doesn't mean more is better.

A common assumption is that shelf-stable fermented foods are automatically useless because all the beneficial microbes must be dead. Some shelf-stable products are pasteurized and no longer contain live microbes, but that doesn't make them completely worthless. They may still provide acidity and flavor. Some refrigerated products can also vary in how many live microbes they actually contain. The cleaner rule is this, if your goal is live fermentation-associated microbes, favor refrigerated, unpasteurized products with simple ingredients. If your goal is mainly flavor and acidity, pasteurized products may still have a place.

KIMCHI: THE MORE COMPLEX FERMENT

Kimchi is a more complex fermented vegetable food. It's usually made from cabbage and other vegetables with ingredients such as garlic, ginger, and red pepper. Its fermentation creates organic acids and a changing microbial environment, which is why it has received attention in gut-health discussions.

The practical value of kimchi in a ketovore framework isn't that it acts like medicine. It's that it offers acidity, spice, strong flavor, and fermented-food character in a very small portion. Garlic and ginger contain compounds that can affect microbes in laboratory settings, and they also influence kimchi's flavor and fermentation process. But the cleaner claim is this, these ingredients contribute to the flavor and fermentation profile of kimchi. Kimchi shouldn't be treated like a targeted antimicrobial treatment.

This is also where labels matter. Many commercial kimchi products include added sugar, rice flour, or other ingredients that make them less useful in a low-carbohydrate framework. That doesn't mean all commercial kimchi is a problem, but it does mean ingredient discipline matters. If you're using kimchi as a condiment inside an animal-based structure, the cleaner and simpler the ingredient list, the better.

The Real Use Case

Both sauerkraut and kimchi make the most sense when used in small amounts alongside meat-based meals. Think spoonfuls, not servings. Their job is to add acidity, flavor contrast, and possibly some fermentation-related benefits without becoming the center of the plate. In that role, they may improve consistency and meal enjoyment, especially for someone who wants a small amount of variety without sliding back into plant-heavy eating.

If the fermented condiment becomes an excuse to rebuild bowls, wraps, and layered vegetable-heavy meals, then the role of the food has changed. The right question isn't, "is kimchi healthy?" The right question is, "does this small amount improve the framework or pull me away from it?"

Fermented vegetables may reduce some plant-related burden and provide flavor, acidity, and fermentation-related benefits, but they work best in a ketovore framework when treated as optional condiments rather than major food groups.

THE STRATEGY: CONDIMENT, NOT MAIN COURSE

The secret to using fermented foods successfully in a ketovore framework is restraint. Fermented foods work best when they stay small, strategic, and clearly secondary to the animal-food foundation. The moment they start becoming side dishes, snack foods, or a new category of "healthy" eating to build meals around, they stop functioning like tools and start becoming drift.

A forkful of sauerkraut, a few spoonfuls of kefir, or a small portion of plain Greek yogurt may be enough to test tolerance, add acidity, or create a little contrast alongside a rich meat-based meal. You aren't trying to fill your stomach with fermented foods. You're testing whether a small amount improves the system without adding new friction. Fermented foods may influence the gut environment, but the benefits aren't guaranteed, they don't require large portions, and they vary by product and person.

- **One Forkful Is Plenty**

That line captures the discipline of the whole strategy. A small serving is often enough to see whether a food improves flavor, digestion, or consistency without turning it into a larger variable. This matters because fermented foods are still foods, not medicine. More isn't automatically better. In fact, larger portions often make it harder to tell whether the ferment is helping, whether the amount is too much, or whether the body is reacting to the underlying dairy or vegetable itself.

- **Balance the Richness**

This is one of the most practical uses of fermented foods. The acidity of sauerkraut, the tang of kefir, or the sourness of unsweetened yogurt can cut through the heaviness of fatty meat and make a meal feel more balanced without adding much carbohydrate. That culinary effect matters more than people admit. Long-term consistency is often helped by small amounts of contrast.

- **Listen to the Feedback**

If fermented dairy makes you feel bloated, gassy, congested, or inflamed, don't rush to one automatic explanation. It might be lactose. It might be casein. It might be dairy sensitivity in general. Fermented dairy often contains less lactose than regular milk, and some people tolerate kefir or yogurt better than milk. But "better tolerated" doesn't mean universally tolerated. If your body reacts poorly, the theory doesn't matter. The food isn't working for you.

The same caution applies to plant ferments. Gas or bloating after kimchi or sauerkraut doesn't automatically mean SIBO, or Small Intestinal Bacterial Overgrowth. SIBO can cause bloating, gas, abdominal pressure, discomfort, and changes in bowel habits, but those symptoms can also come from many other digestive issues. Fermented foods may bother some people because of histamine sensitivity, portion size, the vegetable itself, added ingredients, or the current state of the gut. Don't over diagnose yourself based on one reaction. Pay attention, simplify, and test carefully.

- **Return to Baseline When Necessary**

If fermented foods start creating digestive noise, the smartest move is often to simplify again. Return to a stricter baseline for a period of time and let the system quiet down. A short stretch of very simple carnivore eating can help you separate the signal from the static. Returning to a strict Lion-style approach for about two weeks can be a reasonable practical reset, not because fourteen days is magic, but because a simpler baseline makes patterns easier to see. Once symptoms settle, reintroduce carefully and in very small amounts.

The Bigger Lesson

Fermented foods work best when they behave like seasoning, not sustenance. Their job is to support the framework, not compete with it. If a spoonful of sauerkraut, a small serving of kefir, or a little plain Greek yogurt improves the meal and causes no problems, it may have a place. If it creates bloating, cravings, congestion, digestive noise, or confusion, remove it and return to the foundation.

FERMENTED JUICE: THE LOW-RESIDUE OPTION

For some people, the best way to use fermented plants isn't to eat the vegetables at all, but to use the juice. A small amount of brine from sauerkraut, kimchi or your home made fermented foods can provide the sourness, salt, and fermented character of the food without the fiber, bulk, and plant matter that may irritate a sensitive digestive system. This makes fermented juice a useful low-residue option for the person who wants a small amount of fermentation support without turning the condiment into a side dish.

This approach is especially practical for people who find that the vegetables themselves cause bloating, fullness, or unnecessary digestive noise. In those cases, the brine may be a cleaner way to test tolerance. You're getting a concentrated, flavorful liquid that carries the acidic and fermented qualities of the food while leaving behind most of the plant material. In a ketovore framework, that's often smarter than forcing down forkfuls of cabbage or kimchi simply because they're considered "healthy."

The key is dose. Fermented juice should be treated like a tonic, not a beverage. A teaspoon to a tablespoon alongside a meat-heavy meal is often enough to see whether it adds something useful. It can be sipped slowly, used almost like a palate cleanser, or added to a bite of fatty meat to cut through the richness. The purpose isn't hydration. The purpose is controlled exposure.

This can also be a helpful stepping stone. Some people tolerate the juice well but react poorly to the plant solids. Others discover that even the juice creates digestive symptoms, which is useful information. In either case, the body is giving feedback. The juice allows you to test the ferment with less plant burden, less fiber, and less room for overeating.

There are a few cautions. First, many fermented brines are very salty. That may be useful in some situations, but it can become excessive in large amounts. Second, flavored commercial products may contain added sugars, spices, preservatives, or other ingredients that make the juice less useful in a carnivore-based framework. Third, if you react badly to histamine-rich foods or fermented foods in general, the juice may still create symptoms even without the vegetables themselves. Removing the solids doesn't guarantee tolerance.

The practical rule is simple, if fermented vegetables feel like too much, start with the juice. Use a very small amount, pair it with a meat-based meal, and let your own response determine whether it belongs in the protocol. If it adds flavor and digestive ease without creating bloating, cravings, or irritation, it may be a useful tool. If it adds noise, it doesn't earn its place.

Bottom line: Fermented juice can be a cleaner, lower-residue way to experiment with plant ferments. It keeps the dose small, the plant burden low, and the feedback easier to read.

If fermented vegetables are too much, the brine may be enough. Sometimes the smartest way to use a food is to take its signal without taking its bulk.

SUMMARY OF CHAPTER 9

In this chapter, we added one final fine-tuning tool to the framework, fermentation. But we did so with the proper hierarchy in place. Fermented foods aren't the foundation of a carnivore or ketovore way of eating. They're optional tools. The foundation remains ruminant meat, animal fat, and the simple animal-based meals that have anchored the entire book. Fermentation, when used well, doesn't replace that foundation. It adds a small layer of strategic support for the person who tolerates it and benefits from it.

We explored both animal-based and plant-based ferments through that lens. Fermented dairy, such as kefir and Greek yogurt, was presented as a potentially useful option for people who already tolerate dairy well and want a fermented food that fits more naturally into an animal-based structure. Fermented vegetables, such as sauerkraut and kimchi, were treated more cautiously, as optional condiments rather than side dishes or health foods to build meals around. In both cases, the rule remained the same.

These foods should stay small, controlled, and secondary to the meat-based framework. Their value depends entirely on whether they improve the system without adding cravings, bloating, digestive problems, or dietary drift.

We also refined the strategy further by introducing fermented juice as a lower-residue option. For some people, using a small amount of brine from sauerkraut or kimchi makes more sense than eating the plant matter itself. This allows them to experiment with the acidic and fermented qualities of the food while leaving behind most of the fiber and bulk of the vegetables. In that sense, fermented juice can serve as an even more controlled tool, something closer to a tonic than a food. It reinforces the larger lesson of the chapter, fermentation works best when it's treated with precision, not enthusiasm.

That led to the most important takeaway of all, condiments, not the main course. Whether the ferment is dairy-based, plant-based, or simply the juice from a fermented vegetable, it should remain in its proper place. These foods aren't there to rebuild complexity or slowly pull the diet back toward old patterns. They're there, if used at all, to serve the framework without competing with it. If they improve flavor, consistency, or digestion without creating noise, they may have earned a place. If they destabilize the system, they should be removed without sentiment.

The takeaway from Chapter 9 is simple, fermentation is a tool, not a requirement. It may help some people fine-tune the system, but only when used in small, intentional amounts and always in service of the animal-food foundation. At this stage, success no longer comes from adding more. It comes from judging more clearly what deserves to stay.

By the end of this chapter, the hierarchy should be unmistakable. Meat remains the foundation. Ferments are controlled variables. Use them only if they improve the system without reshaping it and keep them small enough that they season the framework instead of competing with it.

CONCLUSION

If you have made it this far, you understand this was never just about food.

Food was the starting point. The real lesson was clarity. It was about removing enough noise to hear your body again. It was about learning the difference between real hunger and cravings, between adaptation and warning signs, between useful stress and stress that slowly breaks you down.

The modern world trains people to ignore their own signals. We eat all day and still feel hungry. We chase caffeine, snacks, screens, and stimulation and call it energy. We live in comfort but become weaker, tired, stiff, and disconnected. Then we are told health has to be complicated. This approach goes the other direction.

That is the real value of this framework. It is not about being perfect. It is not about joining a diet tribe. It is not about proving discipline to anyone else. It is about building a way of life that gives you a better life You now know how to build your diet on a solid foundation, how to be flexible without losing control, how to spot the difference between useful tools and traps, and how to work with your body instead of fighting it all the time.

Some people will stay very strict. Some people will be flexible. Some people will need more structure in the beginning and more options later. The details matter, but they are not the main point. The main point is simple: health improves when you remove what keeps causing problems, give your body what it handles well, and stay consistent long enough for the pattern to show itself.

For me, this meant getting my energy back. It meant fewer cravings, clearer thinking, better sleep, and a level of stability I had not felt in years. It meant no longer feeling controlled by appetite, fatigue, and constant thoughts about food. It meant taking responsibility for my health in a way that was simple, direct, measurable, and hard to fake.

This book does not promise perfection, because life does not offer perfection. What it gives you is a framework. A way to quiet food noise. A way to make better decisions. A way to trust your body's feedback again.

But the work does not become real because you reached the last page. It becomes real when you stop waiting for permission and start living in a way that makes you stronger, clearer, and more capable.

Healing does not always happen in a straight line. Your energy may rise, then dip. Your digestion may improve, then shift again. The scale may move quickly, then stall. That does not automatically mean the plan has failed. Biology is not always clean or predictable. A body shaped by years of processed food, hunger, poor sleep, stress, and confusion does not become calm overnight. It changes through repetition. It responds to patterns. It often improves in ways that are real before they are obvious.

So do not demand a perfect timeline. Stay with the process long enough to see the results.

The map is in your hands now.

Eat real food. Drink water. Use salt wisely.
Lift heavy things. Sprint when your body is ready.
Walk in the sun. Sleep hard.
Pay attention. Adjust honestly. Stay free.

Stay the course.

— Clinton

GLOSSARY OF TERMS

This glossary defines the key terms used throughout the book. Some come from nutrition science, physiology, metabolism, and medicine. Others are practical terms commonly used in carnivore, ketovore, ketogenic, and low-carbohydrate communities.

The goal isn't to turn this into a medical dictionary. The goal is to make the language of this book easier to understand. These definitions explain how each term is used inside this framework, not every possible way the term may appear in a textbook or clinical setting.

Use this section as a quick reference whenever a term needs clarification or read it straight through as a condensed review of the ideas this book is built on.

Adaptation Phase: The transition period when the body adjusts to lower carbohydrate intake and begins relying more on fat and ketones for fuel. This phase can include changes in fluid balance, sodium needs, digestion, appetite, sleep, and exercise performance. It may feel unstable before it feels smooth.

ADF — Alternate-Day Fasting: A more aggressive fasting strategy that alternates normal eating days with days of full fasting or very low-calorie intake. It can be useful in selected cases, but it isn't a beginner protocol and shouldn't be treated as automatically better than gentler fasting schedules.

Allulose: A low-calorie rare sugar used by some people as a temporary sweetener during transition. It appears to have a much smaller blood sugar effect than regular sugar, but it should be treated as a tactical crutch rather than a permanent staple.

Antinutrients: Biologically active compounds found in plants that can reduce mineral absorption or create digestive or immune irritation in some people. Examples include phytates, oxalates, lectins, and glycoalkaloids. Their effects depend on the food, preparation method, dose, and individual tolerance.

Autophagy: A normal cellular cleanup process where damaged proteins and worn-out cell parts are broken down and reused. Fasting is one condition that may support autophagy-related pathways, but the exact timing and strength of that effect in humans are still being studied.

Bioavailability: How well a nutrient can be absorbed and used by the body. Animal foods are often valued because they provide highly usable nutrients such as heme iron, vitamin B12, retinol, and complete amino acids.

Carnivore-Adjacent: See Ketovore.

Carnivore Diet: A simple animal-based way of eating built around meat, eggs, fish, and animal fats. It removes plant foods, processed foods, sugar, seed oils, and modern additives so the body has fewer things to react to. The goal is to provide highly usable nutrition while making hunger, digestion, energy, and metabolism easier to manage. At its core, carnivore isn't only about restriction. It's about returning to the foods humans have relied on for strength, survival, and nourishment for generations.

Circadian Rhythm: The body's internal twenty-four-hour clock. It helps regulate cortisol, melatonin, insulin sensitivity, body temperature, hunger signals, immune activity, and sleep quality. Light is one of the main signals that sets this rhythm. Morning sunlight tells the body the day has started. Evening darkness tells the body it's time to wind down and recover. When circadian rhythm is aligned, many systems work better. When it's disrupted by too little daylight, too much artificial light at night, or irregular sleep timing, energy, recovery, metabolism, and hormone balance can suffer. In this framework, circadian alignment is treated as an environmental input that matters alongside food quality.

Clean Fast: A fasting period that includes only non-caloric or nearly non-caloric inputs such as water, plain tea, black coffee, salt, or electrolytes. It's the clearest version of fasting from a meal-timing perspective.

Dawn Phenomenon: An early-morning rise in blood glucose caused by hormones such as cortisol and growth hormone, which signal the liver to release fuel as the body prepares to wake up and move. On a low-carb or carnivore diet, this can become more noticeable because blood sugar may be steadier the rest of the day.

Dirty Fast: A fasting period that includes small calorie additions, such as heavy cream or bone broth. It may still help some people stay consistent, but it isn't the same physiological state as a stricter clean fast.

Electrolytes: Charged minerals such as sodium, potassium, and magnesium that help support nerve function, muscle contraction, hydration, and blood volume. On low-carbohydrate diets, sodium and fluid losses can increase, which makes electrolyte awareness especially important during the transition phase.

Fat Adaptation: A metabolic adjustment where the body becomes better at using dietary fat and stored body fat for energy. This doesn't mean carbohydrates become unusable. It means the body becomes less dependent on frequent glucose intake.

Food Noise: The constant mental chatter about food, cravings, and eating that shows up even when you aren't truly hungry. Food noise can feel like a constant preoccupation with what to eat, when to eat, how much to eat, or whether you should eat at all. Reducing food noise is one of the major practical benefits many people notice when they move away from processed foods and build meals around protein and fat.

Gluconeogenesis — GNG: A normal process where the liver makes glucose from non-carbohydrate sources, such as amino acids and glycerol. This helps supply glucose to the tissues that still need it, even when dietary carbohydrate intake is very low.

Hyper-Carnivorous: A term used in ecology and anthropology to describe a dietary pattern where most food comes from animal sources. In discussions of human evolution, it's often used to describe the high position on the food chain seen in some ancient human populations, especially during parts of the Pleistocene.

Insulin Resistance: A condition where the body's cells don't respond to insulin as well as they should. This can lead to higher insulin levels, poorer blood sugar control, and broader metabolic problems. Insulin resistance is strongly associated with obesity, metabolic syndrome, and type 2 diabetes.

Intermittent Fasting — IF: A meal-timing strategy that creates periods of eating and periods without food. It doesn't decide what you eat, it only changes when you eat. Its usefulness depends on context, recovery, consistency, and whether it makes your life more stable instead of more stressful.

Keto Flu / Carnivore Flu: A group of early transition symptoms that can include headache, fatigue, cramps, irritability, brain fog, and disrupted sleep. These symptoms are often linked to fluid and electrolyte shifts, lower sodium levels, and the stress of adapting to very low carbohydrate intake.

Ketones: Energy-rich molecules made by the liver, especially when carbohydrate intake is low and fat use increases. Ketones can serve as an alternative fuel source for the brain, heart, and other tissues.

Ketovore: A high-fat, animal-based way of eating that combines the foundation of carnivore with some of the flexibility of a ketogenic diet. The main focus remains fatty meats and other animal foods, but this approach allows small, strategic additions such as fermented foods, low-toxicity whole-food plants, and whole-food fats. It can be an easier transition into an animal-based lifestyle because it allows more variety while still keeping carbohydrates low. The goal is to keep the body using fat for fuel while giving the person more flexibility and options.

Lean Mass Hyper-Responder — LMHR: A pattern seen in some lean, insulin-sensitive people on carbohydrate-restricted diets who develop very high LDL-C along with low triglycerides and high HDL-C. This is a real observed pattern, but what it means for long-term heart health is still debated.

Lion Diet: The strictest form of carnivore. It usually includes only ruminant meat, salt, and water, meaning foods like beef, bison, lamb, deer, or elk. The purpose is to make food as simple as possible. When almost everything is removed, it becomes easier to see what the body reacts to and what it handles well. This approach is often used by people dealing with serious food sensitivities, digestive problems, autoimmune symptoms, skin issues, or metabolic problems. It isn't meant to be fancy. It's meant to be simple, clear, and easy to track.

Lipid Panel: A common blood test that usually includes total cholesterol, LDL-C, HDL-C, and triglycerides. In a low-carb or carnivore context, interpretation should focus on the overall pattern rather than one isolated number.

Low Energy Availability: A state where energy intake is too low for the body's needs after exercise and daily life are accounted for. It can impair recovery, thyroid function, mood, performance, and, especially in women, menstrual function.

Low-Residue Diet: A diet that leaves relatively little undigested material to form stool. Animal-based diets often produce less stool volume than fiber-heavy diets. This can reduce bowel frequency without automatically meaning constipation.

Maillard Reaction: The browning reaction that happens when proteins and sugars on the surface of food are exposed to enough heat. This creates the savory flavor and crust that make seared meat more satisfying.

Metabolic Flexibility: The body's ability to switch between fuel sources, including glucose and fat, depending on food intake, activity, and demand. Better metabolic flexibility generally reflects a more adaptable system.

Net Carbs: A labeling concept that subtracts certain fibers and sugar alcohols from total carbohydrates. It can be useful in some situations, but it doesn't perfectly predict blood sugar response, cravings, or digestive tolerance.

OMAD — One Meal a Day: A fasting pattern where all daily food is eaten in one meal. It can work for some experienced people, but it isn't automatically better than a wider eating window. It can also become under-eating in disguise.

Oxalates: Compounds found in certain plant foods that can contribute to kidney stone risk in susceptible people. They may also create problems for some individuals depending on intake, tolerance, and overall health context.

Plateau: A period where visible progress, especially scale weight, appears to stop. Plateaus may reflect water retention, stress, poor recovery, inconsistent adherence, reduced activity, or true metabolic adaptation. A plateau doesn't automatically mean the plan has failed.

Protein Poisoning / Rabbit Starvation: A state associated with eating very lean diets that provide too much protein relative to fat and total energy. It can lead to fatigue, poor fullness, digestive distress, and low energy when the body isn't getting enough fat or total fuel.

Ruminant: An animal with a multi-chambered stomach that ferments plant material before absorption. Examples include cattle, sheep, goats, bison, deer, and elk. Because of this fermentation process, ruminant meat usually has a more stable fat profile than meat from animals like pigs or chickens.

Satiety: The feeling of being full, satisfied, and nourished enough that the drive to keep eating goes down. In this framework, high satiety is one of the main advantages of meals built around enough protein and fat.

Seed Oils: Industrial oils such as soybean, corn, sunflower, safflower, cottonseed, and canola oil. These oils are high in polyunsaturated fats and are commonly used in ultra-processed foods. In this book, they're treated as lower-priority fats because they're highly processed and less stable under heat than more saturated animal fats.

SIBO — Small Intestinal Bacterial Overgrowth: A condition where too many bacteria are present in the small intestine. It's often associated with bloating, gas, abdominal discomfort, and changes in bowel habits. These symptoms overlap with many other digestive problems, so SIBO shouldn't be casually self-diagnosed from one food reaction.

Sleep: The main recovery period of the twenty-four-hour cycle. During sleep, the body repairs tissue, regulates hormone rhythms, restores the nervous system, and processes the demands of the day. In a carnivore framework, sleep isn't treated as passive rest. It's the recovery environment where food, training, light, and fasting deliver much of their benefit. Poor sleep can worsen hunger, cravings, blood sugar control, recovery, and metabolic stability. Some people experience lighter or disrupted sleep during the early transition phase but sleep often improves as the body adapts.

Standard Carnivore: The most sustainable baseline version of carnivore for many people. It usually uses ruminant meat as the foundation, along with other animal foods such as eggs, seafood, poultry, pork, and animal fats, depending on tolerance and goals.

TG/HDL Ratio: The ratio of triglycerides to HDL cholesterol. It's often used as a rough marker of metabolic health and insulin sensitivity, especially in low-carb discussions. It can be useful, but it should be interpreted as part of a larger pattern rather than treated as a final verdict by itself.

Time-Restricted Eating — TRE: A form of intermittent fasting that limits eating to a specific daily window, such as 12:12, 16:8, or 20:4. It focuses on daily meal timing rather than prolonged multi-day fasting.

Ultra-Processed Foods — UPFs: Industrial food products made by breaking whole foods into parts, modifying them, and combining them with additives. They often contain ingredients not commonly found in a home kitchen, such as high-fructose corn syrup, hydrogenated oils, artificial colors, gums, flavoring agents, and preservatives. They're usually designed for convenience, long shelf life, strong flavor, and easy overeating.

Wolff's Law: The principle that bone adapts to the force placed on it. In simple terms, bone becomes stronger when it's exposed to appropriate stress through lifting, impact, and movement.

FREQUENTLY ASKED QUESTIONS

Questions are unavoidable when you move against conventional nutrition advice. Some will come from other people. Many will come from old messaging already living in your own mind. This section gives you clear, practical answers without turning every concern into a debate.

Safety & Long-Term Health

Q: Is this safe to do long term?

For many people, an animal-based diet built around real, unprocessed foods can work well and be sustainable. The real question is not whether the diet looks different from what most people eat. The real question is whether it helps you feel and function better over time. Pay attention to the basics: your energy, digestion, hunger, cravings, body composition, sleep, mood, and bloodwork. Long-term success depends on how well the diet is built, how your body responds, and whether you are honest about the results. Do not defend the diet just because you want it to work. Watch the feedback. Adjust when needed. Use common sense.

Q: What about nutrient deficiencies? Don't I need vegetables for vitamins?

Not necessarily. Animal foods provide many essential nutrients in highly usable forms, including protein, iron, zinc, vitamin B12, and retinol. A well-structured carnivore or animal-based diet can be very nutrient-dense, especially when it includes ruminant meat, animal fat, eggs if tolerated, seafood, and strategic use of organ meats if desired. Vegetables aren't the only path to micronutrients.

Q: Do I need organ meats to do this correctly?

No. Organ meats are useful tools, not requirements. They can increase nutrient density, especially liver, but many people do well without forcing large amounts of them. Use them strategically if they help. Don't turn them into a stumbling block if they don't.

Q: Isn't this too restrictive?

It can feel restrictive at first, especially if you're used to constant variety and highly processed food. But many people eventually find that simplicity feels less restrictive than living in a constant cycle of cravings, food decisions, and unstable hunger. What looks restrictive from the outside may feel clarifying from the inside.

Metabolism & Bloodwork

Q: Will my cholesterol increase?

It might. Some people see LDL rise on low-carb or carnivore diets, while triglycerides often fall and HDL often rises. That's why one number shouldn't be treated like a final verdict. Look at the broader pattern, not just one marker by itself.

Q: What numbers matter most on a lipid panel?

Total cholesterol is usually the least useful number on its own. Triglycerides, HDL, and the triglyceride-to-HDL ratio often give a better first look at metabolic health. If LDL rises significantly, context matters even more. In that case, it may be worth looking at non-HDL cholesterol, apoB if available, blood pressure, waist size, blood sugar control, family history, and, when appropriate, imaging such as a coronary artery calcium score.

Q: Why is my fasting blood sugar higher in the morning?

That can be the dawn phenomenon, which is an early-morning rise in glucose driven by hormones that help prepare the body to wake up and move. On carnivore, this may look more obvious because blood sugar may be steadier the rest of the day. A mildly higher morning reading isn't automatically a problem, especially if the broader pattern is stable.

Q: Should I be checking ketones?

Not unless there's a specific reason. Ketones can be useful in some situations, but chasing ketone numbers isn't the same as improving health. Better fullness, steadier energy, cleaner digestion, reduced cravings, better sleep, a shrinking waist, and improved body composition are usually more useful signals than test strips.

Watch the real-world results first. Is your waist going down? Are you losing body fat? Is your appetite calmer? Is your energy steadier? If those things are improving, ketone testing may not add much. If progress stalls, symptoms are confusing, or you simply want more data, then checking ketones can be useful. Just don't confuse measuring ketones with making progress.

DIGESTION & SATIETY

Q: What about fiber? Won't I get constipated?

Not automatically. Animal-based diets produce less residue, which means less stool volume and sometimes less frequent bowel movements. That isn't the same thing as painful constipation. If there's no bloating, pain, or straining, going less often may simply reflect a lower-residue diet.

Q: What if I get diarrhea in the first few weeks?

That's common enough to expect during transition. Many people tolerate rendered liquid fat poorly at first, especially when they consume too much of it too quickly. If this happens, simplify your meals, reduce free liquid fat temporarily, favor fat attached to meat instead, and give the digestive system time to adapt.

Q: Why am I less hungry than I used to be?

Because meals built around enough protein and fat are often more satisfying than processed mixed diets. One of the biggest shifts on carnivore is that hunger can become quieter, steadier, and less urgent.

Q: How much should I eat?

Enough to feel properly fed and satisfied. In the beginning, under-eating is one of the most common mistakes. If you're constantly cold, weak, irritable, sleeping poorly, or hungry soon after eating, the issue may not be the diet itself. It may be that you're simply not eating enough, not eating enough fat, or not getting enough salt and fluids.

Fasting & Meal Timing

Q: Do I need to do intermittent fasting for carnivore to work?

No. Fasting is optional. It often becomes easier once satiety improves, but it isn't required for success. It should function as a tool, not an identity.

Q: What fasting schedule should I start with?

Start with the least aggressive schedule that feels natural. For many people, that means a simple overnight fast, 12:12, or 16:8. More aggressive approaches should be earned, not forced.

Q: What if fasting makes me feel worse?

Then it's probably too aggressive for your current state. If fasting leaves you depleted, cold, under-recovered, irritable, or obsessed with food, the answer is usually not more fasting. It's less fasting, more support, more stability, and less stress.

Q: Is "dirty fasting" okay?

It can be, depending on your goal. Water, plain tea, black coffee, salt, and electrolytes create the cleanest fasting conditions. Small additions like cream or broth may still help with consistency, but they aren't the same physiologically as a stricter fast. Use them carefully. They may be useful as a transition tool, but they shouldn't be treated like a loophole.

SLEEP

Q: Why has my sleep gotten worse since I started carnivore?

Sleep disruption during the first two to four weeks of carnivore can happen. It doesn't automatically mean the diet is failing. As insulin levels shift, electrolytes change, and the nervous system adjusts to a new fuel environment, sleep can temporarily feel different. You may fall asleep easily but wake up in the middle of the night. You may have unusually vivid dreams. You may feel like your sleep is lighter or less restful than usual.

Adequate sodium, magnesium glycinate at night, and enough total food can help some people during this phase. For many people, sleep improves as adaptation progresses.

Q: Will my sleep improve on carnivore long term?

For many people, yes. Once the body adapts, sleep may become deeper and more consistent. One reason may be better nighttime energy stability. Some people wake at two or three in the morning because the body is responding to a drop in blood sugar and a rise in stress hormones. On a fat-adapted, low-carbohydrate diet, some people experience fewer of those nighttime disruptions.

That doesn't mean carnivore fixes sleep for everyone. Sleep is affected by light exposure, stress, caffeine, alcohol, meal timing, sleep apnea, training load, and the sleep environment. But many people do report that sleep becomes more stable once full adaptation arrives. The full explanation is in Chapter 5.

Q: Can sleep affect my results on carnivore?

Yes. Poor sleep can work against your results in a major way. It can increase hunger, worsen cravings, reduce insulin sensitivity, interfere with recovery, and keep stress hormones elevated when the body should be winding down. In practical terms, chronically poor sleep can fight against many of the metabolic improvements this framework is designed to support.

You can eat well and still feel driven to overeat, store fat, and recover poorly if sleep is consistently inadequate. Protect sleep with the same seriousness you protect your food.

Women, Hormones, Pregnancy, and Children

Q: Can women do carnivore?

Yes, but implementation matters. Women often need to pay closer attention to total food intake, recovery, stress, sleep, and fasting. The issue is usually not carnivore itself. The issue is often under-eating, overtraining, poor sleep, or stacking too many stressors at once.

Q: Can children eat this way?

Children can benefit from nutrient-dense animal foods, but strictness should be handled carefully. Growing bodies need enough energy, protein, fat, minerals, and overall nutrition. For many families, a meat-first or animal-based ketovore approach that minimizes sugar, seed oils, and ultra-processed foods is more practical than forcing a rigid adult protocol onto a child.

Performance & Exercise

Q: Can I build muscle on carnivore?

Yes. Meat provides high-quality protein with the full amino acid profile needed to support muscle growth. The bigger questions are whether you're eating enough, recovering well, sleeping enough, and training properly. Muscle doesn't grow from protein alone. It grows from protein plus resistance training plus recovery.

Q: Why does my performance feel worse at first?

Many people experience an adaptive dip during the early transition. Explosive output, repeated intervals, and gym sharpness may temporarily decline while the body adjusts to a different fuel mix. This is usually a phase, not a final verdict. Support the transition with enough food, enough fat, enough sodium, good hydration, and intelligent training.

Q: Will endurance improve?

Possibly, but not automatically. Some people report steadier long-duration energy once they adapt, but performance depends on the sport, intensity, adaptation time, sleep, recovery, and overall execution. Better fat oxidation doesn't guarantee better results in every athletic setting.

BUDGET, PRACTICALITY, AND SOCIAL LIFE

Q: Is carnivore too expensive?

Not necessarily. Carnivore becomes expensive when people insist on premium steaks, specialty products, and convenience foods. It becomes much more practical when built around ground beef, cheaper ruminant cuts, bulk buying, eggs if tolerated, and simple meal structure.

Q: Do I need perfect sourcing for this to work?

No. Better sourcing is better when you can afford it, but don't let perfect become the enemy of effectiveness. The jump from processed junk food to conventional beef is much bigger than the jump from conventional beef to ideal beef. Consistency matters more than perfectionism.

Q: What if I "cheat"?

One off-plan meal isn't a failure. The bigger danger is turning one mistake into a spiral. Return to simple animal food at the next meal and move on without drama. Don't punish yourself with starvation, excessive fasting, or guilt. Just return to the framework.

Q: How do I handle social situations?

Keep it simple and brief. A line such as, "I'm doing a strict elimination diet right now," usually works better than trying to educate the whole table. Social pressure is often a bigger problem than hunger, so decide your standard before you arrive. Know what you'll order, have your answer ready, and don't turn every meal into a debate.

Ferments, Bridge Foods, and Gray Areas

Q: Do I need fermented foods for gut health?

No. Fermented foods are optional tools, not foundational foods. Some people do well with kefir, Greek yogurt, sauerkraut, kimchi, or even just fermented brine. Others do better without them.

Q: Are low-carb "keto" products okay?

Usually, they aren't worth it, especially during transition. Many of these products keep the old reward loop alive and preserve the psychology of processed food under a different label. Simplicity usually works better than substitutes.

Q: Can I use allulose or other sweeteners?

Possibly, but treat them as temporary tools, not permanent fixtures. A tactical sweetener may help some people avoid a full rebound into junk food during transition, but the long-term goal is a quieter palate, not a more clever way to keep sweetness central.

Q: Can I use fermented juice instead of eating fermented vegetables?

Yes. For some people, a small amount of fermented brine is a cleaner, lower-residue option than eating the plant matter itself. It allows a small test of tolerance without adding as much fiber, bulk, or plant load.

RED FLAGS

Q: When should I stop guessing and get medical help?

Severe weakness, fainting, persistent vomiting, blood in the stool, chest pain, major unintended weight loss, or clearly worsening blood sugar control aren't things to explain away as "adaptation." The same applies to persistent loss of a menstrual cycle, severe hair shedding, or profound ongoing fatigue. At that point, medical evaluation matters more than dietary troubleshooting. When in doubt, get medical help.

Q: When should I be concerned about sleep problems specifically?

Mild sleep disruption in the first two to four weeks can happen during transition. But if sleep remains severely fragmented beyond the first month, if you're waking repeatedly every night with a racing heart, if you're snoring heavily and waking unrefreshed despite enough time in bed, or if sleep problems are getting worse instead of better, those patterns deserve medical evaluation. Sleep apnea in particular is closely linked with excess body weight, insulin resistance, and metabolic dysfunction, and it deserves proper assessment instead of assuming adaptation will fix it.

REFERENCES & FURTHER READING

The books and media listed below are included as resources for further exploration, not as blanket endorsements of every claim or recommendation made by their authors. These works have influenced my thinking or contributed meaningfully to the broader discussion around nutrition, metabolism, and human performance.

Their inclusion doesn't imply their endorsement, affiliation, or recommendation of this book or its conclusions. The perspectives presented in this book are my own, and responsibility for their interpretation and application rests solely with me as the author.

FOUNDATIONAL BOOKS

- Baker, Dr. Shawn. *The Carnivore Diet*. Victory Belt Publishing, 2019.
- Berry, Dr. Ken. *Lies My Doctor Told Me: Medical Myths That Can Harm Your Health*. Victory Belt Publishing, 2019

- Bikman, Benjamin. PHD. *Why We Get Sick: The Hidden Epidemic at the Root of Most Chronic Disease, and How to Fight It*. BenBella Books, 2020.
- Saladino, Dr. Paul. *The Carnivore Code: Unlocking the Secrets to Optimal Health by Returning to Our Ancestral Diet*. Houghton Mifflin Harcourt, 2020.
- Sisson, Mark. *The Primal Blueprint*. Primal Nutrition, 2009.
- Teicholz, Nina. *The Big Fat Surprise: Why Butter, Meat, and Cheese Belong in a Healthy Diet*. Simon & Schuster, 2014.

EDUCATIONAL MEDIA & ONGOING COMMENTARY

- **Dr. Shawn Baker, MD.** Educational media and commentary on carnivore nutrition, performance, and metabolic health.
- **Dr. Ken Berry, MD.** Educational media focused on medicine, low-carbohydrate nutrition, and carnivore principles. Proper Human Diet.

- **Benjamin Bikman, PhD.** Educational media and interviews focused on insulin resistance and metabolic health.
- **Dr. Paul Saladino, MD.** Educational media and commentary on animal-based nutrition and ancestral health.
- **Dr. Anthony Chaffee, MD.** Educational media and commentary on plant-free nutrition and human evolution.
- **Dr. Annette Bosworth, MD (Dr. Boz).** Educational media focused on ketogenic nutrition, (Sardine) fasting, and metabolic health.
- **Dr. Sean O'Mara, MD, JD.** Commentary on fermented foods, body composition, visceral fat, and metabolic function.

Suggested Reader Approach

Use these resources as starting points for deeper study, not as substitutes for your own judgment. Some of these authors agree with each other. Some don't. Some take stronger positions than this book does. That's fine. The purpose of this list isn't to hand you a finished worldview. It's to give you a map so you can keep exploring with more context, sharper judgment, and better questions.

Page Intentionally left Blank.

CITATIONS:

American Diabetes Association. (n.d.). Low Blood Glucose (Hypoglycemia). https://diabetes.org/living-with-diabetes/hypoglycemia-low-blood-glucose. Accessed June 22, 2026.

Budoff, M., Manubolu, V. S., Kinninger, A., Norwitz, N. G., Feldman, D., Wood, T. R., Fialkow, J., Cury, R., Feldman, T., & Nasir, K. (2024). Carbohydrate restriction-induced elevations in LDL-cholesterol and atherosclerosis: The KETO trial. *JACC: Advances*, *3*(8), 101109. https://doi.org/10.1016/j.jacadv.2024.101109

Bull, F. C., Al-Ansari, S. S., Biddle, S., Borodulin, K., Buman, M. P., Cardon, G., et al. (2020). World Health Organization 2020 guidelines on physical activity and sedentary behaviour. British Journal of Sports Medicine, 54(24), 1451–1462. https://doi.org/10.1136/bjsports-2020-102955

de Cabo, R., & Mattson, M. P. (2019). Effects of intermittent fasting on health, aging, and disease. The New England Journal of Medicine, 381(26), 2541–2551. https://doi.org/10.1056/NEJMra1905136

Dimidi, E., Cox, S. R., Rossi, M., & Whelan, K. (2019). Fermented foods: Definitions and characteristics, impact on the gut microbiota and effects on gastrointestinal health and disease. Nutrients, 11(8), 1806. https://doi.org/10.3390/nu11081806

Feingold, K. R. (2025). Guidelines for the Management of Dyslipidemia. In Endotext. MDText.com, Inc.

Food and Agriculture Organization of the United Nations. (2013). Dietary protein quality evaluation in human nutrition: Report of an FAO Expert Consultation. FAO Food and Nutrition Paper, 92, 1–66.

Garegnani, L. I., Oltra, G., Ivaldi, D., Burgos, M. A., Andrenacci, P. J., Rico, S., Boyd, M., Radler, D., Escobar Liquitay, C. M., & Madrid, E. (2026). Intermittent fasting for adults with overweight or obesity. Cochrane Database of Systematic Reviews, 2026(2), CD015610. https://doi.org/10.1002/14651858.CD015610.pub2

Gordon, C. M., Ackerman, K. E., Berga, S. L., Kaplan, J. R., Mastorakos, G., Misra, M., Murad, M. H., Santoro, N. F., & Warren, M. P. (2017). Functional hypothalamic amenorrhea: An Endocrine Society Clinical Practice Guideline. The Journal of Clinical Endocrinology & Metabolism, 102(5), 1413–1439. https://doi.org/10.1210/jc.2017-00131

Hall, K. D., Ayuketah, A., Brychta, R., Cai, H., Cassimatis, T., Chen, K. Y., et al. (2019). Ultra-processed diets cause excess calorie intake and weight gain: An inpatient randomized controlled trial of ad libitum food intake. Cell Metabolism, 30(1), 67–77.e3. https://doi.org/10.1016/j.cmet.2019.05.008

Hudgel, D. W., Patel, S. R., Ahasic, A. M., Bartlett, S. J., Bessesen, D. H., Coaker, M. A., et al. (2018). The role of weight management in the treatment of adult obstructive sleep apnea: An official American Thoracic Society clinical practice guideline. American Journal of Respiratory and Critical Care Medicine, 198(6), e70–e87. https://doi.org/10.1164/rccm.201807-1326ST

Institute of Medicine. (2005). Dietary Reference Intakes for Energy, Carbohydrate, Fiber, Fat, Fatty Acids, Cholesterol, Protein, and Amino Acids. National Academies Press. https://doi.org/10.17226/10490

Jelleyman, C., Yates, T., O'Donovan, G., Gray, L. J., King, J. A., Khunti, K., & Davies, M. J. (2015). The effects of high-intensity interval training on glucose regulation and insulin resistance: A meta-analysis. Obesity Reviews, 16(11), 942–961. https://doi.org/10.1111/obr.12317

Kohanmoo, A., Faghih, S., & Akhlaghi, M. (2020). Effect of short- and long-term protein consumption on appetite and appetite-regulating gastrointestinal hormones: A systematic review and meta-analysis of randomized controlled trials. Physiology & Behavior, 226, 113123.

Kohrt, W. M., Bloomfield, S. A., Little, K. D., Nelson, M. E., & Yingling, V. R. (2004). American College of Sports Medicine Position Stand: Physical activity and bone health. Medicine & Science in Sports & Exercise, 36(11), 1985–1996. https://doi.org/10.1249/01.MSS.0000142662.21767.58

Mizushima, N., & Komatsu, M. (2011). Autophagy: Renovation of cells and tissues. Cell, 147(4), 728–741. https://doi.org/10.1016/j.cell.2011.10.026

National Center for Home Food Preservation. (n.d.). General Information on Fermenting. University of Georgia. https://nchfp.uga.edu/how/ferment/general-information-on-fermenting/general-information-on-fermenting/. Accessed June 22, 2026.

National Institute of Diabetes and Digestive and Kidney Diseases. (2025). Lactose Intolerance. https://www.niddk.nih.gov/health-information/digestive-diseases/lactose-intolerance. Accessed June 22, 2026.

National Institutes of Health, Office of Dietary Supplements. (2025). Vitamin D: Fact Sheet for Health Professionals. https://ods.od.nih.gov/factsheets/VitaminD-HealthProfessional/. Accessed June 22, 2026.

Özlek, B. (2026). Reassessing LDL-cholesterol elevations in lean-mass hyper-responders: Clinical significance and unresolved questions. *European Journal of Preventive Cardiology*, zwag038. https://doi.org/10.1093/eurjpc/zwag038

Soto-Mota, A., Norwitz, N. G., Manubolu, V. S., Kinninger, A., Wood, T. R., Earls, J., Feldman, D., & Budoff, M. (2025).

Plaque begets plaque, ApoB does not: Longitudinal data from the KETO-CTA trial. *JACC: Advances*, *4*(5), 101686. https://doi.org/10.1016/j.jacadv.2025.101686

Spiegel, K., Tasali, E., Penev, P., & Van Cauter, E. (2004). Brief communication: Sleep curtailment in healthy young men is associated with decreased leptin levels, elevated ghrelin levels, and increased hunger and appetite. Annals of Internal Medicine, 141(11), 846–850.

StatPearls. (2025). The Ketogenic Diet: Clinical Applications, Evidence-based Indications, and Implementation. StatPearls Publishing.

Sutton, E. F., Beyl, R., Early, K. S., Cefalu, W. T., Ravussin, E., & Peterson, C. M. (2018). Early time-restricted feeding improves insulin sensitivity, blood pressure, and oxidative stress even without weight loss in men with prediabetes. Cell Metabolism, 27(6), 1212–1221.e3. https://doi.org/10.1016/j.cmet.2018.04.010

Tähkämö, L., Partonen, T., & Pesonen, A.-K. (2019). Systematic review of light exposure impact on human circadian rhythm. Chronobiology International, 36(2), 151–170. https://doi.org/10.1080/07420528.2018.1527773

Tani, Y., Tokuda, M., Nishimoto, N., Yokoi, H., & Izumori, K. (2023). Allulose for the attenuation of postprandial blood glucose levels in healthy humans: A systematic review and meta-analysis. PLOS ONE, 18(4), e0281150. https://doi.org/10.1371/journal.pone.0281150

U.S. Department of Agriculture, Agricultural Research Service. (n.d.). FoodData Central. https://fdc.nal.usda.gov/. Accessed June 22, 2026.

U.S. Department of Agriculture, Food Safety and Inspection Service. (n.d.). Safe Minimum Internal Temperature Chart. https://www.fsis.usda.gov/food-safety/safe-food-handling-and-preparation/food-safety-basics/safe-temperature-chart. Accessed June 22, 2026.

U.S. Food and Drug Administration. (2018). Enjoying Homemade Ice Cream without the Risk of Salmonella Infection. https://www.fda.gov/food/buy-store-serve-safe-food/enjoying-homemade-ice-cream-without-risk-salmonella-infection. Accessed June 22, 2026.

Wastyk, H. C., Fragiadakis, G. K., Perelman, D., Dahan, D., Merrill, B. D., Yu, F. B., et al. (2021). Gut-microbiota-targeted diets modulate human immune status. Cell, 184(16), 4137–4153.e14. https://doi.org/10.1016/j.cell.2021.06.019

Yang, J., Wang, H.-P., Zhou, L., & Xu, C.-F. (2012). Effect of dietary fiber on constipation: A meta-analysis. World Journal of Gastroenterology, 18(48), 7378–7383. https://doi.org/10.3748/wjg.v18.i48.7378

ABOUT THE AUTHOR

I was born in the early 1970s and grew up in West Texas during the 1970s and 1980s.

Like most kids back then, I ate the standard American diet. By the time I was eight years old, I was already dealing with hypoglycemia. I learned early what it felt like for blood sugar to crash, for energy to disappear, and for feeling "off" to be treated as normal.

Health problems came slowly at first, then all at once. Arthritis in my back, neck, and hands. Years of NSAIDs and steroid injections. In 2017, I was dealing with premature ventricular contractions, sleep apnea, and an A1C drifting into prediabetic territory. Pain, fatigue, and instability became normal life.

In 2019, after watching The Game Changers, I switched to a vegan diet. At first, things looked better on paper, lower total cholesterol and weight loss. But over time, I gained the weight back. My triglycerides climbed to 158. My HDL stayed in the high 30s. My blood sugar became harder to control, and I found myself needing to eat every couple of hours just to function. I remember thinking, "Our ancestors didn't live this way. This doesn't make sense. What would they have eaten for all of this to make sense?"

That question changed everything.

In January 2024, after digging into the research myself, I transitioned to a low-carbohydrate carnivore lifestyle. The adjustment wasn't easy. Sugar withdrawal was real. Electrolytes mattered more than I ever imagined. It took months, not weeks, but slowly my system stabilized.

Today, I eat once or twice a day without thinking about it. My energy is steady, and my blood sugar no longer crashes. My HDL has gone up to almost 60, and my triglycerides have come down to 95. The pain that once required constant medical intervention is now manageable. My asthma is under control. I went from 240 pounds to under 200, not just through willpower, but by removing what didn't belong.

This book isn't about ideology. It's about paying attention. It's about questioning assumptions that don't hold up under lived experience. It's about taking responsibility for your own health in a world that profits from confusion.

I'm not here to convince anyone. I'm here to share what worked for me when everything else failed.

Stay Connected. Join the Carnivore Uncomplicated Newsletter

Get simple carnivore tips, practical health lessons, book updates, and no-nonsense guidance from Clinton Scitern, author of Carnivore Uncomplicated.

www.clintonscitern.com

YouTube channel:

www.youtube.com/@clintonscitern

Before you close this book and step back into real life, I want to give you something simple to help you start.

Download your **FREE QUICK START BONUS** here:

www.carnivoreuncomplicated.com

To get the most out of this book, grab the companion journal, Carnivore Uncomplicated 30-Day Reset Journal, and use it to track your food, energy, cravings, sleep, movement, and progress during your reset.

www.ingramcontent.com/pod-product-compliance
Lightning Source LLC
LaVergne TN
LVHW052037200926
848481LV00005B/1704
* 9 7 9 8 9 9 6 5 5 9 3 0 5 *